AYURVEDA & IMMORTALITY

AYURVEDA
& IMMORTALITY

Scott Treadway Ph.D. 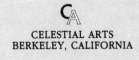 Linda Treadway Ph.D.

CELESTIAL ARTS
BERKELEY, CALIFORNIA

Excerpts from *The Great Secret* by Maurice Maeterlinck reprinted with permission of E.P. Dutton and Company, New York.

Selections from the translation of the *Charaka Samhita,* edited by P.M. Mehta, reprinted with gracious permission of the Honorable Secretary of the Shree Gulabkunverba Ayurvedic Society, Jamnagar, India.

"That Nature is a Heraclitean Fire and of the Comfort of the Resurrection" by Gerard Manley Hopkins reprinted with permission from Little, Brown and Company, Boston.

"The Tridosha Questionnaire" reprinted with permission from Sattva Foundation, Fairfield, Iowa.

Selection *The Pain Game* by C. Norman Shealy, M.D. reprinted with permission from Celestial Arts Press, Berkeley, California.

Selections from the *Berkeley Holistic Health Center Handbook* reprinted with permission of Armand Brent.

Scientific research on Ayurveda reprinted with permission from Dr. Robert Keith Wallace, Dr. David Orme-Johnson, and Dr. Robert Schneider.

A NOTE OF CAUTION

This book presents advanced and enlightened ideas about the traditions surrounding health care. These ideas are presented for your consideration and should be discussed with your physician or health care professional. *This material is meant to enhance your well being and is in no way intended as a substitute for medical care.*

Celestial Arts
P.O. Box 7327
Berkeley, California 94707

Cover and interior design by Ken Scott
Typography by HMS Typography
Printed and bound at Consolidated Printers, Berkeley, California

Library of Congress Cataloging-in-Publication Data

Treadway, Linda.
    Ayurveda and immortality.

    1. Medicine, Ayurvedic.   I. Treadway, Scott.
II. Title.
R606.T74   1986   610   85-28965
ISBN 0-89087-457-3

Made in the United States of America

10 9 8 7 6 5 4 3 2 1 — 9291 90 89 88 87 86

First Printing, 1986

DEDICATION

This book on the great science of Ayurveda is dedicated to His Divinity, Shri Swami Brahmananda Saraswati, Bhagwan Shankaracharya of Jyotir Math, Himalayas.

ACKNOWLEDGEMENTS

To the Founder of the Maharishi Technology of the Unified Field, and to all of its many research scientists and Siddha technologists all over the world, our gratitude and most sincere thanks.

To Celestial Arts Press, of Berkeley, California, for professionalism, vision, and valor.

TABLE OF CONTENTS

TABLE OF CHARTS

FOREWORD

Ayurveda is an ancient science of life and health that reveals to us the scientific means to fulfill the aspirations of both individuals and societies which seek ideal health and longevity. Ayurveda is a holistic system of perfect health which can be fully appreciated by medical scientists as well as lay persons.

Those of us who work in preventive and orthomolecular medicine see daily the lack of awareness which forces medical institutions to function as disease-oriented entities. There is generally more concern about treating the disease rather than preventing it. Ayurveda is health-oriented and offers us a unique understanding of how imbalances develop and how they can be prevented and also how disease is cured.

The preventive approach of Ayurveda is in keeping with our concerns as physicians to guide our patients to the ability to develop an invincible immune system. This system of medicine has the capacity to create an ideal society of happy, healthy individuals who can live long enough to enjoy all the beauty that life has to offer.

This elegant and literate volume introduces the main concepts of Ayurveda in a clear and comprehensive manner. Scott and Linda Treadway are exceptional Vedic scholars with over twenty years of intimate experience with the technology of the unified field and are uniquely qualified as path-cutters in the modern rediscovery of Ayurveda. They have clarified for all readers the main concerns of Ayurveda and have focused their attention on the vedic techniques for prevention of disease through diet and purification, as well as development of the immune system through herbal food supplements and the regular practice of meditation. The profound knowledge described in this book can provide an invaluable direction for improved health management.

Scott and Linda Treadway are well versed in Ayurvedic medical principles and in its emphasis on the development of consciousness as a key element in balancing the physiology. Their appreciation of the goals of Ayurveda and the impact it can have on Western medicine is scholarly, scientific and profound. With this invaluable book we are now beginning to tap the vast potential of Ayurvedic wisdom.

—Michael L. Gerber, M.D.
President, Orthomolecular Medical Society, 1984, 1985
Former Board Member, The American Academy of
Medical Preventics

—

PREFACE

It is a great pleasure for us to be able to share the knowledge that we have gathered over the twenty-year period of our continued fascination with the beauty of the Vedic science, which includes Ayurveda, the indigenous medical system of India.

Ayurvedic medicine has its roots in the *Samhita*, or the totality of natural law, as found in Vedic literature. In any study of Vedic science, primary emphasis must be placed on the wholeness of Vedic knowledge and its ability to make relevant connections to all other fields of knowledge. Vedic science in general is the basis for understanding the knowledge found in the specialized Ayurvedic literature. Our explanation of Ayurveda as a healing science continually refers to that concept of wholeness which is the hallmark of Vedic science.

We were fortunate enough to attend the thirty-three lectures on Vedic science given by His Holiness Maharishi Mahesh Yogi at Maharishi European Research University in 1972. These lectures on Vedic science were designed to contain all the essential knowledge of the Vedic tradition and to impart that knowledge in a universally comprehensible manner. These lectures, along with Maharishi's other works—*Veda: The Source of the Subtle Science*, and his fine translation and commentary on the *Bhagavad-Gita* (Chapters 1–6)— should be required reading for every Vedic scholar. Maharishi's present work in symposia and lectures on the three-in-one structure of consciousness, and the Technology of the Unified Field™, including the Transcendental Meditation™ and TM Sidhi™ program, constitutes a monumental scientific achievement as a modern interpretation of the most ancient Vedic knowledge that subsequently unifies all disciplines of the physical, biological, and social sciences, as well as those of the humanities.

Because Ayurveda has always dealt with the human mind, body, and consciousness in unity, the researcher is continually brought to an appreciation of its wholeness and perfection as a study; its diversity is eternally reflected against the essential unity of life presented by Vedic science. The immense variety in creation grows out of the nonvariable unity of existence, and the ability to bring all fields of knowledge together is the integrative quality of the unified field from which the multiplicity of creation bursts forth. This makes any student of Vedic science doubly fortunate, for the study itself, when combined with the regular practice of Transcendental Meditation or the TM Sidhi program, then becomes a vital method for integrating consciousness and preserving physical health.

The scientific revival of Ayurveda opens the door to immortality for every individual. The central principle of Ayurveda leads us to experience our own immortal state of pure consciousness, defined by Vedic science as the Self, our essential nature. Maharishi has stated that physical immortality is a scientific reality based upon behavior that is in perfect harmony with the laws of nature. So, in addition to the experience of immortality of consciousness, Ayurveda offers us techniques that can lead us in the direction of perfect health, infinite life extension, and physical immortality. This is indeed a fortunate time in the history of humanity, as it provides us with the fascinating opportunity for the serious pursuit of perfect health.

The *Charaka Samhita*, a Vedic treatise on general medicine, and the *Sushruta Samhita*, a Vedic treatise on surgery and toxicology, are the only two complete primary sources remaining out of six original Ayurvedic *Samhitas* (encyclopedias) known to have existed. In India immediately preceding World War II the Shree Gulabkunverba Ayurvedic Society undertook a new translation of the *Charaka Samhita*. An unfortunate delay occurred during the intervening war years, but with its publication in 1949 the six-volume work became an important and definitive translation. In the 1970s the Chowkhamba Sanskrit Series was published, and included both the *Charaka* and *Sushruta* works. One of the major contributors was Dr. V.B. Dash, a commentator of great ability in translating Ayurvedic literature. Dr. Dash has also published several other valuable works on Ayurveda including his doctoral dissertation, *Tibetan Medicine, with Special Reference to the Yoga Sa'taka of Nagarjuna.*

In general, native Indian authors writing in English give the most lucid explanations of this complex subject to the student of Ayurveda. Two of the best Indian exponents of Ayurveda currently writing and publishing in English for American readers are Dr. Vasant Lad and Dr. Chandrashekar Thakkur. Rarely do European or American authors duplicate the excellence of their Indian colleagues. One wishes for more publications from practicing American scholars and physicians such as Dr. Archimedes Concon. In his writings, Dr. Concon correctly identifies traditional acupuncture as originally a Vedic art, subsequently passed along with Sanskrit grammar to the Tibetans and then to the Chinese. Dr. Concon's clinical practice combines allopathic medicine and traditional acupuncture, and he has retained the ability to express that fullness of both intellect and spirit that characterizes the best of Eastern thought.

The problem of bridging the cultural gap between practitioners of Ayurvedic Sciences and practitioners of the biological sciences has limited the number of published articles in English on the subject of Ayurveda. Fortunately, His Holiness Maharishi Mahesh Yogi has recently established a great philosophical structure for the correct explication of Ayurvedic knowledge, as well as centers for the practice of Ayurveda throughout the United States and the world. Maharishi has also gathered the greatest experts on Ayurveda from India and the United States to establish a collegium of Ayurvedic knowledge. World-renowned scholars such as Dr. V.M. Dwivedi, Dr. B.D. Triguna and Dr. H.S. Kasture contributed to this great revival of practical knowledge. Valuable and original research now being conducted will demonstrate the supreme value of Ayurveda to this and future generations.

After a thorough review of the extant literature in English on Ayurvedic medicine, one is made aware that more works are needed in English that fully express the richness of Vedic science, and can also serve as textbooks for the health practitioner and all readers who desire informed self-sufficiency in personal health care. Though this book focuses on the Ayurvedic sciences of *Rasayana* and *Rasashastra* (and not Ayurvedic diagnostics and advanced dietetics, which we leave to later writings), it is our hope that this work, *Ayurveda and Immortality*, will provide a taste of that potential that is within us all, and point a clear direction toward the richness of life offered by Vedic science, which includes an unparalleled opportunity for perfect health and longevity as well as personal and global peace.

We have used phonetic Sanskrit terminology extensively because the vibratory quality of the Sanskrit language is a powerful educational tool in itself. By reading and understanding these terms, one may come to a powerful subjective and subtle level of communication with the natural laws that underlie the objective and outward phenomena of the healing process. A glossary is included at the end of the book for easy reference.

It is an extraordinary privilege to be able to write about the wholeness of the Vedic tradition, since one cannot write effectively about wholeness unless it is lived. Another challenge is to present complete knowledge while remaining consistent in simplicity.

We very much need to thank our loving family, especially Wayne Wetherbee, and our accomplished and wise colleagues and advisors, Dr. Caroline Shrodes, Dr. Paul Kapiloff, Dr. Robert Schneider, Dr. Willis Harman, Dr. Rhoda Orme-Johnson, Dr. David Orme-Johnson, Dr. Robert Keith Wallace, Samantha Wallace and our personal physicians David Walker and Dr. Michael Gerber for their generous support during the writing of this work.

Scott Treadway
Linda Treadway
Fairfield, Iowa

AYURVEDA & IMMORTALITY

C H A P T E R   1

INTRODUCTION TO VEDIC SCIENCE

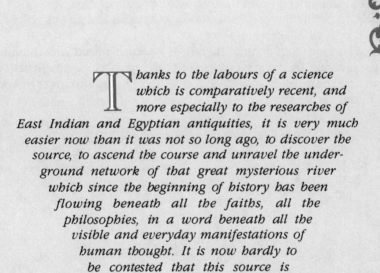

Thanks to the labours of a science which is comparatively recent, and more especially to the researches of East Indian and Egyptian antiquities, it is very much easier now than it was not so long ago, to discover the source, to ascend the course and unravel the underground network of that great mysterious river which since the beginning of history has been flowing beneath all the faiths, all the philosophies, in a word beneath all the visible and everyday manifestations of human thought. It is now hardly to be contested that this source is to be found in ancient India.

Maurice Maeterlinck
THE GREAT SECRET

The word *Veda* comes from the Sanskrit word *vid,* to know. *Veda* means knowledge, pure knowledge or pure consciousness. The ancient East Indian documents known as the four *Vedas* concern themselves with the most fundamental relationships between nature and consciousness. For many years the *Vedas* were looked upon simply as ancient ritual, history, or naive poetry. But due to the recent work of some great scholars of the *Vedas,* the Vedic literary tradition is now recognized to be a complete and transformative body of knowledge, which may be equally important to experience as to understand intellectually. The *Vedas* can only be completely understood from the state of enlightenment. From that high state of human evolution, one knows the *Vedas* to be the living record of how consciousness moves within itself to give rise to all of creation.

The four main texts of the *Vedas* were organized and compiled in their proper form by the great Indian saint Krishna Dvaipayana (Badarayana) who was given the nickname "Vyasadeva," meaning the arranger or compiler. The four *Vedas* are:

1. *Rig Veda*
2. *Sama Veda*
3. *Yajur Veda*
4. *Atharva Veda*

The *Rig Veda* is the seed of the other three *Vedas.* It contains over a thousand verses and is older and longer than the *Iliad* and *Odyssey* combined. All four *Vedas* have been preserved in an oral tradition, mainly by a group of families descended from the Vedic *rishis* (seers) who originally cognized its verses.

The history of Ayurveda, an aspect of the *Vedas* dealing with health and longevity, extends back to the Vedic period. Ayurveda is one of the *Upa Vedas* (subordinate *Veda*). Ayurveda goes into great detail on the subject of medicine and medical treatment for the establishment of health, longevity, the elimination of disease, and ultimately immortality.

Ayurvedic literature is estimated to have been recorded at least 2000 years before Christ. Ayurveda has existed in India longer than any other system of medicine, and is believed to be the parent of all Oriental medicine and Greek medicine and, subsequently, of all Western medicine.

To understand Vedic science, and Ayurveda as a branch of Vedic science, we must first recognize that the foundation and source of the *Veda* is the *Samhita,* or wholeness, the encyclopedic compendium recording the function of natural law. Both modern science and Vedic science have located the foundation of all the laws of nature in a single unified field. Maharishi

4

Mahesh Yogi equates the unified field with pure consciousness, the simplest state of awareness. This unified field, which has been identified by modern physics as the source of all energy fields and fundamental particles, is the same field experienced by those individuals who meditate daily. One can experience the unified field of immortal being as the Self.

Vedic science is the science of consciousness, a comprehensive explanation of how the unified field appears to diversify into the multiplicity of creation and how that diversity unifies into wholeness again. The three essential aspects of consciousness are known as *rishi* (observer/knower), *chhandas* (observed/known), and *devata* (process of observation or knowing). These three self-referral aspects of the unified field are the three-in-one values, not only of the unified field, which is always awake in the knowledge of its own nature, but also of all other levels of creation. All of life can be understood as functioning within the three-in-one structure of consciousness which is described in detail in the Veda.

The first of the three-in-one values is called the value of *rishi* (knower). This is the awareness of the Self that is the witness or observer of any object of perception or thought. Next in the three-in-one structure is the *chhandas* (object itself) that is observed by the observer: the chair, house, automobile, thought, feeling, action, or any object that we experience. The third aspect of the three-in-one structure is *devata*, the process of observation. Observation proceeds through the intellect, the senses or other mediums of perception (within consciousness). Vedic science defines this three-in-one structure as *samhita*, or wholeness, where the three essential qualities of consciousness, *rishi*, *devata*, and *chhandas*, are unified.

THE THREE-IN-ONE STRUCTURE OF THE UNIFIED FIELD (THE VEDA)

1. *Rishi*	Observer-knower-Self	
2. *Devata*	Process of observation or of gaining knowledge	
3. *Chhandas*	Observed, object of the senses	

This knowledge of the three-in-one structure of the unified field is the science of consciousness. We can say that the reality of the one unified field pervades the conceptual reality of the three-in-one structure (which includes diversity), or we can say that the three-in-one structure exists within the all-pervasive unified field. Whatever we say, the three-in-one reality of diversity is only a *conceptual* reality, a viewpoint upheld by the intellect. The unified field, is always one reality. As a healing science, Ayurveda is based on a continuing acknowledgment of this essential unity.

The unified field is immortal and uncreated, nonconceptualized, pure consciousness, ever the same. Even so, the intellect conceptualizes multiplicity in the unified field. Vedic science demonstrates how the unified field of consciousness seems to become diversified and how that diversity seems to be unified, while the unified field itself remains unchanged. It is the greatness of the *Vedas* that they explain what seems unexplainable.

Ayurveda has not yet been fully understood because the nature of the unified field has not been fully understood. The usual empirical approach of modern science is not able to thoroughly investigate the unified field. In the past, modern science has insisted upon a strong separation of the observer and the observed. This attitude goes against the very nature of understanding the unified field, which is *Samhita* or wholeness. That is why the *Vedas* recommend the practical approach of deep meditation. Deep meditation allows a real experiential understanding of the unified, an experience of the ultimate unity of observer, process of observation, and observed (the three-in-one structure of consciousness). This provides a strong basis for investigating the structures of natural law residing in Ayurveda.

Modern science generally focuses on the objective *(chhandas)* value of life, but modern science is destined to unify with Vedic science. This is because the unified field *(Veda)* is the source of the *chhandas* value, the source of the entire three-in-one structure, and the source of all values, structures and scientific investigations. The *samhita* of the *Veda* (the totality of natural law or wholeness of the *Veda*) is leading modern science to the inevitable conclusion that the consciousness of the observer *(rishi)*, the observed object *(chhandas)*, and the process of observation *(devata)*, cannot be separated if there is to be a complete understanding of the various phenomena of life.

By tradition the *Veda* is considered the primary expression of universal intelligence and a blueprint of the primary impulses of original creation. It is considered the template of universal knowledge in all its aspects—that which holds true for all time and space. In the Vedic tradition, daily meditation is practiced routinely to maintain and cultivate the mind and body so as to experience the infinite nature of pure consciousness. Then, as the individual grows in conscious awareness of the Self, the ability to experience all aspects of one's nature and of the environment increases.

The great Vedic sage Adi Shankara remarked that words do not exist that can adequately describe the grandeur of human consciousness to experience the range of its own intelligence. He suggests that, after fundamental knowledge of the structure of consciousness is gained, it is better to live it than continually to analyze it.

In order to live in good health through the continuous processes of natural evolution, a protective and preventive modality for the culture and maintenance of all aspects of life is required. The science of Ayurveda was revealed to the Vedic seers as a primary means for protecting life so that the

6

individual, supported by a healthy mind and physiology, might have sufficient time and opportunity to evolve into the realization of the unbounded immortal nature of Self and experience all of the possibilities of life.

The next chapter shows how the Vedic *rishis* (scholars) structured the knowledge of the *Veda* into the discipline called *Ayurveda*. We shall see that applying the universal knowledge in the *Veda* maintains and restores individual health so that the primary activity of creation, the evolution of consciousness, may freely take place.

This knowledge is as useful today as when it was first compiled thousands of years ago by the seers of the *Veda*, and for the same universal reasons. We all wish to grow in health and happiness. We all wish to live to see our children's children. These considerations have not changed with time. The history of Ayurveda is the record of how these aspirations were achieved by the Vedic *rishis* and how the systematized knowledge of Ayurveda may prove to be more useful to our technological generation than even we can envision at present.

Ayurveda as a healing art was first remembered (cognized not composed) by Brahma, who taught it to Daksha-Prajapati, who taught it to the Ashwin-kumaras, and they taught it to Indra as they healed him. In the Ayurvedic text known as the *Charaka Samhita,* it is stated that at the end of the Vedic period a great gathering of seers took place at the foot of the Himalaya mountains, and these great sages appointed one of their number, Baradwaja, to learn the knowledge of Ayurveda from Indra. Two direct descendants within this Ayurvedic tradition are Charaka and Sushruta. Both produced Ayurvedic encyclopedias, or *samhitas.* The lore of Ayurveda has been preserved for thousands of years and much of it can now be found in the *Charaka Samhita* or *Sushruta Samhita,* both currently used Ayurvedic texts.

The following is how P.M. Mehta, an editor of the Ayurvedic treastise the *Charaka Samhita* describes the scientific evolution of Ayurveda:

> *Suffice it to know now that from this (Vedic) period we enter upon the variegated scene of the Samhita period or the period of systematic and scientific compilation . . . . At the end of this Vedic age we must place the great congress of sages described in the opening lines of the* Charaka Samhita, *who gathered together to discover the way of healing and long life faced with the undeniable reality of deadly disease and pestilence that snatched away the flower of humanity and made impossible the higher progress and evolution of all life through meditation and thought. With that conference in the Northern Himalayas dawns the scientific age of medicine in India.*

THE UNIVERSAL NATURE OF VEDIC KNOWLEDGE

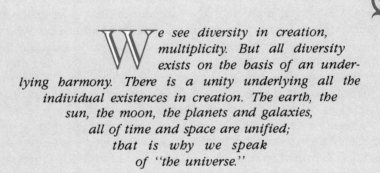

We see diversity in creation, multiplicity. But all diversity exists on the basis of an underlying harmony. There is a unity underlying all the individual existences in creation. The earth, the sun, the moon, the planets and galaxies, all of time and space are unified; that is why we speak of "the universe."

Maharishi Mahesh Yogi

Ayurveda, one of the *Upa Vedas* (subordinate *Veda*), is the knowledge of *ayus*, or life itself. Ayurveda brings us the understanding of balance in nature and in ourselves as a part of nature. Preventing imbalance that leads to aging and death is the primary function and first responsibility of Ayurveda; Ayurvedic medicine is preventive by nature. The second responsibility of Ayurveda is curative, to restore balance where imbalance may have developed.

In the past, Ayurveda has been separated from its roots in the *Veda*. Because of this is has not been universally successful. The present reunification of Ayurveda with the *Samhita* (wholeness or totality of the *Veda*) insures that it will become universally valuable.

The purpose of Ayurveda is to establish or restore balance and harmony in the mind and body, so that wholeness of life can be experienced in a natural state of health. The preventive health procedures of Ayurveda bring about a state of complete balance that is reflected in excellent health and an invincible immune system.

The ultimate purpose of Ayurveda is to allow the individual to rise to the highest state of enlightenment or unity consciousness, a state that exhibits a perfect balance in all aspects of life.

At one time or another, many of us have experienced pure awareness, that crystalline moment of pure consciousness which is the experience of the Self. It is a universal experience and the essence of the universal human condition. For some it occurs regularly in the quietness of meditation or reverie; for others it occurs in the inner silences created by poetry and music; for others visually, in the apprehension of art or nature; for many at the juncture point *(sandhi)* between waking and sleeping, or at the juncture points between night and day (dawn and dusk). Since we have all experienced pure consciousness to some degree, we can relate intimately to the Vedic concept of the universal Self.

According to Vedic science, it is from the Self *(purusha)*, that Nature *(prakriti)* is engendered. The relationship of *purusha* to *prakriti* is one of latent potential energy to manifested energy. *Purusha* gives the impetus and *prakriti* manifests. The mind therefore, is only an expression of the creative capacities of *prakriti*. The senses are a further projection of the creativity of *prakriti* expressed in creation. *Prakriti* manifests itself in various sheaths of matter to create the entire universe. The intellect as part of nature provides us with the sense of conceptual reality by which we understand nature.

At a very subtle stage of evolution, after *prakriti* arises from *purusha*, the three creative tendencies of nature *(gunas)* appear. These creative tendencies of nature are called *sattva, rajas,* and *tamas. Sattva* is the creative impulse of nature, *rajas* is the energetic and maintaining impulse of nature, and *tamas* is the retarding or destructive force of nature. The three *gunas* exist together; the presence of one requires the presence of the others.

According to the *Veda*, these three forces—creation, maintenance, and destruction—are the constituent forces of relative creation, and are born when *prakriti* or nature arises from *purusha* (consciousness). All activity in the universe, including the maintaining of physical health, is carried out by the interplay of these three *gunas*, or tendencies. *Rajo-guna* maintains the process of creation, while *satto-guna* creates a new state and *tamo-guna* destroys the old state. This process allows for movement and change, for the evolution of any system or thing, from one stage to another in an evolutionary direction. The accompanying chart illustrates the relationship of consciousness and nature or *purusha* to *prakriti* and the three *gunas*.

CHART OF THE MANIFESTATION OF CONSCIOUSNESS

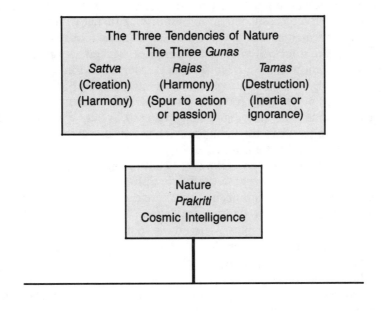

Each of the three *gunas* acts upon the other two and upon itself. The Vedic works called the *Upanishads* describe this constant weaving and winding of the *gunas* and their interaction by saying, "The *gunas* act upon themselves. The Self interacts with itself." *Sattva* has the quality of awareness, purity, relevation and harmony. *Rajas* has the qualities of dynamic movement, creation and passion. *Tamas* has the qualities of inertia and ignorance. In the Ayurvedic system, modes of behavior, choice of diet, and even articles of clothing may be classified as having the quality of one or more of the *gunas*.

For example, milk, clarified butter, grain, fruits and vegetables are considered to be sattvic foods. Hot, spicy, pickled, sour and salty foods are considered to be rajistic foods, and meats, cheeses, fermented and preserved items are considered to be tamasic foods. As seen by the Ayurvedist, all of the *gunas* also effect some physiological change in the human body. Each of the three *gunas* has a physical manifestation. This is called a *dhatu* or *dosha* (meaning "that which supports or governs"). Each *dosha* is divided into two types—that which is grossly perceivable *(sthula)*, and that which is not readily apparent but may be inferred from other manifestations *(shuskma)*.

There are three *doshas*, and a description of their action in dynamic combination is known as the *tridosha* theory. All three *doshas* are normally related to the physiology, although their meaning can be broader. Also, all three *doshas* are universally found in each individual in some state of balance or imbalance. The most basic skill mastered by the Ayurvedist is first to determine the nature of the imbalance, if one exists, and then bring about a state of re-balance of the *doshas*.

Ayurveda contains procedures for eliminating an excessive accumulation of the *doshas* to bring about improved physiological balance, vitality, health and longevity. The eliminated wastes are called *malas*. Chapter Three examines theories of Ayurveda in more detail.

Ancient in its principles, Ayurveda is a complete study of all areas of medicine including diagnosis, medical treatment, surgery, pediatrics, toxicology, rejuvenation, pharmacology, anatomy, physiology, yoga, dietetics, and many other fields of knowledge.

Ayurveda, exists for the preservation of human life and has been practiced in India longer than any other system of medicine. It has become a part of countless other systems of traditional medicine and has greatly influenced the medicine and philosophy of the Greeks (including Hippocrates and Heraclitus), as well as the Tibetans, Chinese, and Hebrews. Ultimately, Ayurveda even influenced the pluralism of the holistic health movement in the United States. Because Ayurveda is based on an understanding of the fundamental nature of life and its inherent relationships, and because it provides solutions for problems inherent in the structure of life itself, Ayurveda is timeless.

Many examples in world literature verify that this universal view remains useful today. One of the most beautiful is the following poem by Gerard Manley Hopkins. Though Christian in context, the poem concerns itself with the relationship between the immortal Self *(purusha)* and the unceasing activity of the three *gunas* born of creation. It is a catalog of concern about the austerity required to retain a unified vision within the confines of nature. It illustrates the dynamic qualities of all three *gunas*, starting with *tamas* and ending with *sattva* and an experience of enlightenment or the immortality of the Self. It provides an example of unity consciousness based on the universal reconciling power of divine intelligence, called by Adi Shankaracharya the faculty of *visakyana*, "an identity of the same substance possessed of seemingly different qualities."

THAT NATURE IS A HERACLITEAN FIRE AND OF THE COMFORT OF THE RESURRECTION

Cloud-puffball, torn tufts, tossed pillows flaunt forth, then chevy on an air-
built thoroughfare: heaven-roysterers, in gay-gangs they throng; they glitter in marches.
Down roughcast, down dazzling whitewash, wherever an elm arches,
Shivelights and shadowtackle in long lashes lace, lance, and pair.
Delightfully the bright wind boisterous ropes, wrestles, beats earth bare
Of yestertempest's creases; in pool and rut peel parches
Squandering ooze to squeezed dough, crust, dust; stanches, starches,
Squadroned masks and manmarks treadmire toil there
Footfretted in it. Million-fueled, nature's bonfire burns on.
But quench her bonniest, dearest to her, her clearest-selved spark
Man, how fast is his firedint, his mark on mind, is gone!
Both are in an unfathomable, all is an enormous dark
Drowned. O pity and indignation! Manshape, that shone
Sheer off, disseveral, a star, death blots black out; nor mark
      Is any of him at all so stark
But vastness blurs and time beats level. Enough! the Resurrection,
A heart's clarion! Away grief's gasping, joyless days, dejection.
      Across my foundering deck shone
A beacon, an eternal beam. Flesh fade, and mortal trash
Fall to the residuary worm; world's wildfire, leave but ash:
      In a flash, at a trumpet crash
I am all at once what Christ is, since he was what I am, and
This Jack, joke, poor potsherd, patch, matchwood, immortal diamond,
      Is immortal diamond.

                                 Gerard Manley Hopkins

The Ayurvedist is trained to live this unity of life and to see each being as unique, as *jivataman,* "immortal living soul" of the *purusha,* and to *evaluate normality only on an individual basis and in a serial manner through time,* since the progress of the evolution of consciousness is affirmed as the primary goal of all life.

CHAPTER 3

SPECIFIC AYURVEDIC THEORIES

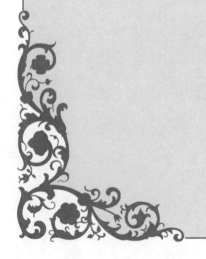

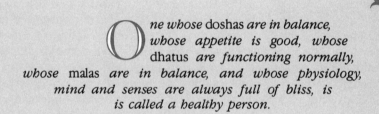

One whose doshas *are in balance,*
whose appetite is good, whose
dhatus *are functioning normally,*
whose malas *are in balance, and whose physiology,*
mind and senses are always full of bliss, is
is called a healthy person.

Sushruta Samhita

Ayurveda, the system of hygiene, dietetics, and medicine developed and perfected in India thousands of years ago, is almost entirely unknown in the West. It truly comprises a great secret, and the teaching of this knowledge will be of inestimable benefit to all humankind. Ayurveda is an entire science of living, perfectly compatible with the popular shift in Western consciousness toward the practice of preventive medicine, holistic health, and optimal nutrition.

According to Ayurvedic theory, the human constitution and all of manifest creation) is composed of five basic elements. These five elements are earth, water, fire, air and space. Ideally, these five basic elements exist in a dynamic harmony, creating life, health, and the perfection of living creation.

At their most subtle stage of manifestation each of the five elements (*mahabhutas*) is endowed with a single quality. In earth, it is solidity; in water, it is liquidity; in fire it is heat; in air it is pressure; and in space it is subtle sound. The five elements correspond to the five senses in human and other living beings. The five material states that correspond to the five elements are: solid, liquid, radiant matter, gaseous matter, and space. In Ayurveda, the five-element theory has been applied to the origin of creation, as well as to human life, to the physiological organization of the human body, and to the curative powers of Ayurvedic treatments, diet regimens, herbal remedies, and food supplements.

Ayurvedist Dr. V.B. Dash gives an example of these five basic elements in physical science. We may conceptualize atomic particles as representing *prithivi* (the earth element) and their cohesion as a function of *jala* (the water element). Energy manifested within and without the atomic field is *agni* (the fire element). Movement of the particles is *vayu* (the air element), and the space through which they move is *akasha*.

Both the objective states of matter and the subjective experiences of the senses arise from *prakriti* (nature) at the level where consciousness manifests into matter and energy. This vital correlation of subjective and objective experience through the mechanisms of consciousness is only now being explored by Western scientists, whereas in Vedic science it has been an accepted fundamental theoretical and philosophical position for thousands of years. All of Eastern thought displays the accepted but usually unspoken connection between the knower, the process of knowing, and the known.

In our sensory experience the five elements (mahabhutas) combine to produce a continuity of sensation. Production of sound comes from space *(akasha)* and the sensation of touch from the air element and space element intermixed. The sense of heat is a mixture of space, air and fire. The water element contains the previous three elements and liquidity, and the solidity of the earth element contains all five.

The *tridosha* theory, which is a principle theory of Ayurveda, holds that each aspect of creation, including human physiology, is constituted from these five basic elements. These five elements combine into three governing factors. These three major governing factors *(doshas)* are named *vata*, *pitta* and *kapha*.

In the theory of the *tridosha*, earth and water elements are combined in a representation of their most common function—as in water moistening earth—and called *kapha dosha*; water and fire combine into a representation of their most common functioning—as in the chemical fire of digestive juices—and called *pitta dosha*; and air and space are combined—as in air moving through space—and are called *vata dosha*.

The *tridosha* theory of the three *doshas*, when applied to human physiology, allows the Ayurvedist to identify and treat each unique and individual body type or constitution. Every individual has a specific balance of *doshas* that is naturally correct according to the original birth constitution. This is called the *prakriti* or constitutional type of the individual. By making a thorough examination of characteristics such as the pulse, body structure, hair, skin, tastes, habits, and other factors, the Ayurvedist will determine the *prakriti* or constitutional type, and will then be able to recommend specific balancing therapies, diets or cures appropriate for that body type.

Prakriti, in the sense of body type, determines what sort of diet, exercise, and life style is appropriate for each individual. Clear information about an individual's constitutional type is essential for any Ayurvedic treatment, since that is what is necessary to bring the individual increased balance, improved health, higher consciousness, longevity, and the prevention of aging, is based on universal knowledge of each individual body type and its unique needs.

To illustrate more clearly the flow of evolution from the unified field to the five elements *(mahabhutas)* and also the relationship of the five elements to the *tridosha* theory of Ayurveda, we offer the accompanying charts. The designation of the five elements is essentially physical, while the *tridosha* theory describes forces responsible for physiological functioning. According to Ayurveda, health is a condition of dynamic balance in the *dhatus*, the tissues that support the body. When the *dhatus* are not balanced they are referred to as *doshas*, which in this sense means "impurity" (from the sanskrit word for fault or break). Some Ayurvedists compare the *doshas* to pools of water that are constantly being filled by the pressures of biological function. Preventive health measures continually "drain" the physiology before the "water" of the *doshas* overflows the container and symptoms of illness or imbalance appear.

19

CHART OF THE MANIFESTATION
OF CONSCIOUSNESS

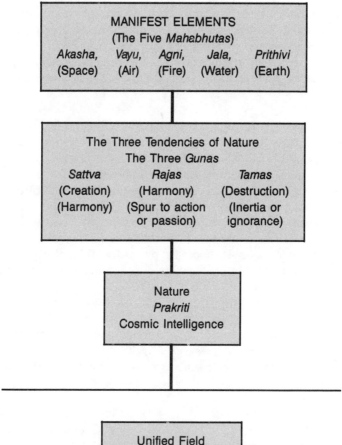

MANIFEST ELEMENTS
(The Five *Mahabhutas*)

Akasha,	*Vayu,*	*Agni,*	*Jala,*	*Prithivi*
(Space)	(Air)	(Fire)	(Water)	(Earth)

The Three Tendencies of Nature
The Three *Gunas*

Sattva	*Rajas*	*Tamas*
(Creation)	(Harmony)	(Destruction)
(Harmony)	(Spur to action or passion)	(Inertia or ignorance)

Nature
Prakriti
Cosmic Intelligence

Unified Field
Purusha
Pure Consciousness
The Self
Immortal

CHART OF THE FIVE ELEMENTS

Element	Corresponds to sense of:	Relates to body as:	Has elemental qualities of:
1. Space *(akasha)*	hearing	ears	non-resistance, softness, lightness, smoothness
2. Air *(vayu)*	touch	skin	dry, cold, rough, light
3. Fire *(agni)*	sight	eyes	warm, active, clear, acid
4. Water *(jala)*	taste	tongue	moist, viscous, cold, soft, slimy
5. Earth *(prithivi)*	smell	nose	heaviness, solidity, slow, bulk, oily, sweet

AYURVEDIC TRIDOSHA THEORY CHART

The three *Doshas*
Vata (a combination of space and air elements)
Pitta (a combination of fire and water elements)
Kapha (a combination of the water and earth elements)

Dosha	Quality	Physiological action on the individual	Psychological action on the individual
Vata	Light, dry, cold, rough, moving, quick, subtle	Nerve functions, motor and sensory, muscular, respiration	activation energy movement
Pitta	Hot, fluid, acid, light	Digestion, sight, metabolic action, thirst and hunger	memory, desire, creativity, joy, chivalry
Kapha	Cold, soft, slow, heavy, unctuous, dull	Lubrication, growth, strength, endurance, potency	friendship, intelligence, generosity, austerity, courage, forgiveness

Upon close scrutiny, it can be seen that the three *doshas—kapha, pitta,* and *vata—*are responsible for the activity and regulation of all physiological processes. In harmony, they are called *dhatus*; when imbalanced, they are called *doshas*, and when excreted, they are called *malas*. (For the sake of clarity and consistency, they are generally called *doshas*.) By balancing the three *doshas* Ayurveda is capable not only of curing the patient but also of refining the individual physiology to smooth the way for higher evolution, enlightenment and, ultimately, immortality.

The *tridosha* theory enables any health practitioner to treat each individual as unique. Even if two people suffer from the same complaint, an Ayurvedist will view them as individuals and often treat them differently. It is said that one should treat a person in whom *vata dosha* predominates as a friend; a person in whom *pitta dosha* predominates as a lover; and a person in whom *kapha dosha* predominates as an opponent. This means that the first type can be gently nudged toward health, the second type needs much reassurance and support during the healing process, and the third type must be firmly reminded to meet the requirements necessary for cure.

In each individual all three *doshas* are present at the time of conception. The predominant *dosha (kapha, pitta, or vata)* forms the major part of the birth constitution, but the remaining *doshas* also help in the initial formation of the physiology. Even though one *dosha* may predominate, the other two will be present to some degree in the physical constitution.

We know that the distinguishing feature of Ayurvedic treatment is its universal nature. Neither in theory nor in fact is there a physical manifestation that cannot be accounted for by the *tridosha* theory. Encompassing all aspects of sensory data, the *tridosha* theory discovers three fundamental types of processes that are responsible for human health. The *Sushruta Samhita* (a treatise on Ayurveda) calls the process of energetic activation *vata*. The activity of producing heat, light, energy, digestion, and transformation is called *pitta*. That process which manifests stability, solidity, and inertia is called *kapha. Vata* comes from the sanskrit *va*, to move; *pitta* comes from the sanskrit *tap*, to produce heat; and *kapha* comes from the sanskrit *shlish*, to join, embrace, or adhere.

The *doshas* manifest in a triplicity just as do the *gunas.* The three *doshas* work in a continuous dynamic harmony to maintain health in the body. They are pervasive in the body and, without adequate prevention, their working inevitably causes impurities to accumulate. Over a twenty-four hour period the *doshas* predominate in turn. Air *(vata)* is preponderant in late afternoon, fire *(pitta)* at noon or midday, and water *(kapha)* in the morning. The cycle repeats itself during the evening, night and pre-dawn hours. The *doshas* are distributed throughout the body. *Vata* below the navel, *pitta* between the navel and the heart, and *kapha* above the heart.

Each of the *doshas* represents a quality of force, a way of manifestation of the laws of nature. Though the Sanskrit word *vata* means "air," the correct conception of the term *vata dosha* is the process of movement or energetic activation. *Kapha* and *pitta* are said to be motionless and require *vata dosha* for activation. Just as air is dry, *vata* is dry, cold, rough, and moving. In the body, *vata* can be thought of as nerve force.

The term *pitta dosha* signifies the force that heats, lights, metabolizes, and transforms. In the body, *pitta* is responsible for digestion and metabolism.

Kapha has been called the primal constituent of the human being, exhibiting a "healthy inert" quality. The force for which it is named is manifested in instinctive behavior, bodily endurance, growth, lubrication of the joints, courage, forgiveness, potency, and cohesion of bodily tissues. *Kapha* is cold, unctuous, and heavy; *pitta* is hot, fluid, and sharp; *Vata* is cold, light, and dry. The eternal interplay among these forces accounts for all types of biological and physiological functions.

A summary of the three basic constitutional types shows them to be distinct and, after some practice, easy to identify. The *tridosha* questionnaire on pages 23–26 will allow you to discover your unique individual body type or *prakriti* according to the *tridosha* theory.

TRIDOSHA QUESTIONNAIRE

TEST INSTRUCTIONS

1. For each category (1–25) on the questionnaire, select the one choice that most closely approximates your individual constitution, either:
- Kapha (water-type)
- Pitta (fire-type)
- Vata (air-type)

Then put a check in the appropriate box. For example, if your response to the first question is *endomorph*, check box 1, column K.

2. When you have finished answering all 25 questions, add the number of check marks in each category and enter the sum in the subtotal boxes.

3. To obtain a percentage ratio of the three elements in your personal constitution, multiply the number of answers in each subtotal box by 4. If you answered all 25 questions, the three percentage figures should add up to 100, and you will have an approximate picture of your unique constitutional type as determined at conception.

4. Conclusion: Usually one element will predominate—that is, will be a larger percentage of the total. In Ayurvedic medicine, this is considered the main constitutional type for diagnosis and treatment of the individual.

Constitutional characteristic	K Kapha	P Pitta	V Vata
1. Body (frame)	Endomorph: broad shoulder/ hips	Mesomorph: medium frame	Ectomorph: narrow hips/ shoulders
2. Weight	Heavy	Neither too thin nor too stout	Slender— tendons show
3. Endurance/ Strength	Good	Moderate	Little
4. Skin texture	Pale, oily, white, moist	Soft, oily, fair, pink, delicate, red	Dry, rough, cool, dark- er com- plexion
5. Skin aging	Smooth, few wrinkles	Freckles, moles, pig- mentation	Dry, flaky, cracked
6. Hair lubrication	Oily	Medium	Dry
7. Hair color	Medium to dark brown, medium blonde	Light brown, red, light blonde	Dark brown to black
8. Hair texture	Straight, thick	Wavy, fine	Curly
9. Digestion/ hunger	Moderate, no exces- sive hunger	Sharp hunger	Irregular or heavy diet, but re- mains thin
10. Teeth	Large, white, resistant to decay	Yellowish, moderate size	Crooked, large, protruding
11. Eyes	Large, blue or brown	Green, gray, hazel	Small, black
12. Elimination	Heavy, slow	Moderate	Tends toward consti- pation

Constitutional characteristic	K Kapha	P Pitta	V Vata
13. Sex drive	Cyclical, infrequent	Moderate	Frequent
14. Physical activity	Avoids exercise, lethargic	Likes regular exercise	Restless, active
15. Mental activity	Calm, steady	Intelligent, aggressive	Restless, active
16. Voice/speech	Harmonious, low-pitched, singing, slow, monotone	Medium-pitched, sharp, laughing, shouting	High-pitched, weeping, vibrato, dissonant
17. Taste/food preference	Dry, low-fat, light, sweet, pungent	Sweet, medium, light, warm, bitter, astringent	Sweet, oily, soupy, heavy, salty
18. Sleep	Easy, deep	Medium, sound	Short, insomnia
19. Memory	Long-term memory	Good, but not prolonged	Short-term memory
20. Financial behavior	Saves money regularly	Saves, but spends on luxury items	Spends money quickly
21. Emotional reaction to stress	Indifference, complacency, withdrawal	Anger, jealousy	Fear, anxiety
22. Dreams	Water, river, ocean, lake, erotic	Struggle, fire, anger, violence, war	Fear, flying, running, jumping
23. Mental pre-disposition	Stable/logical	Judging/artistic	Questioning/theoretician

Constitutional characteristic	K Kapha	P Pitta	V Vata
24. Resting radial pulse/ *quality* (self-diagnostic)	Slow, moves like swan	Moderate, jumps like frog	Thready, slithers like snake
25. Radial pulse/ *quantity* of beats per minute (self-diagnostic)	60–70 beats per minute	70–80 beats per minute	80–100 + beats per minute

Subtotal K _____   Subtotal P _____   Subtotal V _____

X4 = _____ %   X4 = _____ %   X4 = _____ %

GRAND TOTAL _____ (express as a percentage)

The grand total is the sum of the subtotals and should equal 100 (100% expressed as a percentage) if you answered all 25 questions.

Based on my highest subtotal score, my approximate body type is (circle one):

> *Kapha* type (highest subtotal score—K)
> *Pitta* type (highest subtotal score—P)
> *Vata* type (highest subtotal score—V)

©Copyright 1984, by Sattva Foundation

Each constitutional type displays all three *dosha* qualities to some degree. At the time of conception our physical constitution reflects a unique combination of the *tridosha*. According to the Ayurvedic texts the properties of the *kapha* type are: pale, heavy, cold, smooth, polished, soft, majestic, and slow, as well as sweet, delicate, and slippery. This constitutional type has soft, silky, oily, fine skin. The body is muscular, symmetrical, and fleshy. The *kapha*-type person is fond of the sweet tastes and, since *kapha* is cold in action, the *kapha* type likes foods that are hot both in temperature and in seasoning. *Kapha* types should avoid fatty foods and oils, as well as dairy products. *Kapha* persons are slow to anger and slow to forget.

The properties of the *vata* type with some exceptions are opposite those of the *kapha type*. The *vata* person tends to act, and react, much more quickly. Movement is characteristic of the *vata* person. The physique is dry, light, mobile, cold and hard, and the body is uniformly slender. The constitution is dry because of the predominance of air. The personality is quick in all things: to love, to forget, to digest, and to move on. Often an excess of *vata* or air is associated with nervousness or neurological disorders. This constitutional type should avoid all drugs and use diet and other natural means to achieve maximum health and longevity.

In the *pitta* constitution the fire element predominates. Often artistic in temperament, this body type tends to think in creative ways. The person in whom the fire element predominates is moderate in build, neither short nor tall, neither heavy nor thin. The qualities of *pitta* are hot and slightly oily. This constitutional type often has problems with thinning hair or premature greyness. Freckles, moles, and skin disorders are also associated with an excess of *pitta dosha*.

The three constitutional types are partially recognized in America as the physiological types of endomorph, mesomorph and ectomorph, as designated by American psychologist William Sheldon. However, Ayurveda provides levels of classification more profound and sophisticated than Sheldon's system. The key to health and longevity is a constant balancing of the *doshas* according to individual body type. The constitutional makeup of all people contain all three *doshas* to some degree.

According to Ayurvedic theory, the six tastes found in all foods also have a significant effect on the balance of the *doshas*. Most foods have a variety of tastes, but one or two predominate. The sweet, sour, salty, pungent, bitter, and astringent tastes affect the *doshas*, either balancing or aggravating them, depending on the body type.

Following is a list of some common foods with their predominating taste and how the tastes affect the *doshas*. Also included are suggested diets for the three basic body types, *vata*, *pitta* and *kapha*. Please note that these diets are only suggestions and should be individually modified. Most body types are not 100 percent *vata*, *pitta* or *kapha*, but usually contain some amounts of the other two qualities.

27

THE TASTES IN FOOD
AND THEIR EFFECT ON THE DOSHAS

The Six Tastes	Common foods that contain these tastes
Sweet	sugar, cream, milk, ghee, (clarified butter), butter, rice, wheat, grapes, cherries, berries
Salty	salt and excessively salty foods
Sour	lemon, other citrus, yoghurt, cheeses, vinegar
Bitter	coffee, spinach and other leafy green vegetables, turmeric
Pungent	black pepper, ginger, cumin, chili, spicy foods
Astringent	beans, some green vegetables, beans

HOW SOME COMBINED TASTES
AFFECT THE DOSHAS

Sweet, sour, salty	Increases *kapha*, decreases *vata*
Pungent, bitter, astringent	Increases *vata*, decreases *kapha*
Pungent, sour, salty	Increases *pitta*
Sweet, bitter, astringent	Decreases *pitta*

Food qualities can also be classified as:

1. Heavy, oily (or moist) foods
2. Light or dry foods
3. Hot or cold (in temperature) foods

Examples of these food qualities are:

Heavy/oily   Milk, butter, ghee, fatty foods, wheat products, oils, cheese, yogurt, cream, nuts, banana, rice, dried fruits

Light/dry   Corn, millet, oats, barley, beans, fresh fruits

Hot or cold Any food or drink

28

These qualities of food generally effect the *doshas* as follows:

Heavy/oily foods	Increase *kapha*, decrease *vata*
Light/dry foods	Increase *vata*, decrease *kapha*
Hot (in temperature) foods	Increase *pitta*
Cold (in temperature) foods	Decrease *pitta*

Because diet is a major means of affecting the balance of the *doshas*, it is suggested that when eating the atmosphere be peaceful and the food be balanced to include all six tastes. Very cold or iced beverages (and food) can interfere with digestion and are to be avoided. Eat only when the previous meal has been completely digested, and rest briefly after the meal. A small amount of liquid, except for milk, may be consumed with the meal. Milk can be drunk alone or with sweet foods or cereals. Large amounts of fluid before, during, or after meals is not recommended.

In Ayurveda, some food combinations are discouraged. For example, a combination of ghee or butter in equal proportion to honey should be avoided, as should cooked honey in any amount. The combination of fish with milk, honey, radish, or sprouted grains is not recommended, nor is milk with radish, garlic, or liquor.

The *doshas* tend to be prominent or aggravated in their seasons. In the United States, the *kapha* season generally begins the first of spring (March through June), *pitta* season begins in summer (July to October), and *vata* season is fall and winter (November through February). Some Ayurvedists believe, however, that winter is *kapha* season and spring is the season in which *kapha* and *pitta* are combined. As a general rule, Ayurveda suggests that foods be taken seasonally to counter-balance the seasonal effect on the *doshas*. Very generally speaking, this means that in winter, when *vata* is aggravated, fewer *vata*-increasing foods should be taken; in summer, fewer *pitta*-increasing foods; in spring, fewer *kapha*-increasing foods.

SUGGESTED DIET FOR *VATA DOSHA*

This body type should eat breakfast and have small light meals throughout the day. *Vata* people do well to avoid foods that are dry or bitter. Sweet and hot foods are good for them. All dairy products are recommended; Ayurvedic herbs are available to correct milk allergies. *Vata* types need to add more oily and sweet foods and sour and salty tastes to the diet. They should drink warm or hot water and use spices such as cinnamon, cardamom, cumin, ginger, salt, cloves, mustard, and licorice. Nuts and nut butters of all kinds are beneficial.

SUGGESTED FOODS

Vegetables	Fruits	Dairy	Grains	Proteins
yams	grapes	all	wheat	fish
potatoes	avocados		short-grain	fowl
sweet	peaches		brown rice	(light
carrots	cherries		basmati rice	meat)
beets	plums			eggs
asparagus	mangos			(fried or
onions	papayas			scrambled)
red cabbage	figs			
cooked	melons			
vegetables	raspberries			
	blueberries			
	strawberries			
	pineapples			
	bananas			
	oranges			

Vata types should avoid foods suggested in *kapha* and *pitta* diets.

> Note: *Vata dosha* is aggravated in fall and winter.
> Increase warm milk, hot water, and oily foods during fall and winter season.

SUGGESTED DIET FOR *PITTA DOSHA*

The *Pitta* constitutional type should eat breakfast, preferably grains, fruits and some dairy products. This body type should avoid chilies, egg yolk, nuts, honey, hot spices, and very hot drinks. If indigestion occurs, lemon juice in water is a cooling drink. *Pitta* types should add cool foods and liquids, sweet, bitter, and astringent tastes. They should avoid honey and sour-tasting foods, such as yoghurt, pickles and aged cheese. Avoid spices except cinnamon, lemon, coriander, cardamom, and black pepper.

SUGGESTED FOODS

Vegetables	Fruits	Dairy	Grains	Proteins
asparagus	cherries	butter	wheat	chicken
cabbage	green grapes	milk	basmati	turkey
potatoes	plums	ghee	rice	soybean
cucumbers	melons		barley	products
zucchini	sweet, ripe			
broccoli	pineapples			
cauliflower	(ripe)			
sprouts	pears			
lettuce	figs			
celery	coconut			
leafy	mangos			
vegetables				

Pitta types should avoid foods suggested in *kapha* and *vata* diets.

> Note: *Pitta dosha* is aggravated in summer, therefore be sure to increase cooling foods and drinks.

31

SUGGESTED DIET FOR *KAPHA DOSHA*

This body type should avoid eating before at least 10 A.M., should avoid sugar, fats, wheat, dairy products, salt, and add lighter, drier foods. *Kapha* types should not eat after the sun has set, especially moist foods such as watermelon and ice cream. The evening meal should be lighter and drier than lunch, which should be the largest meal of the day. *Kapha* types must avoid iced or cold drinks and substitute warm drinks. They should avoid large quantities of food, and over indulgence in the sweet, salty, and sour tastes. Fasting one day a week as a means of weight control and health maintenance is recommended for healthy *kapha* types.

SUGGESTED FOODS

Vegetables	Fruits	Grains	Meats
raw vegetables/ salads	apples	rye	chicken
squash	pears	corn	turkey
onions	cranberries	barley	eggs
potatoes	kiwi fruit	polenta	(not fried
carrots	persimmons	buckwheat	or
cauliflower	pomegranates	small amount	scrambled)
okra		of rice	
artichokes		millet	
asparagus		beans	
lettuce			
beets			
cabbage			
sprouts			
chilies			
radishes			
green peppers			
spinach			
swiss chard			
bok choy			
celery			
broccoli			
sprouts			

Kapha types should avoid foods suggested in *vata* and *pitta* diet.

Note: *Kapha dosha* is aggravated in the spring. At that time decrease the size of meals and increase low-fat, high-fiber foods.

32

Nutritionally, the Ayurvedic approach works through specific procedures for preventing the accumulation of bodily impurities *doshas* through appropriate diet and herbal food supplements for each individual body type. The Ayurvedic approach brings about balance through comprehensive instructions about nutrition, as well as daily and seasonal routines, and personal hygiene. The primary Ayurvedic approach to mental hygiene is through the daily practice of meditation or yoga.

When looking at an individual, the Ayurvedic physician sees the whole person including the immortal Self. This is very different from the traditional Western approach. The Ayurvedic physician conceptualizes the individual as potentially in perfect balance and perfect health. Ayurveda is designed to prevent an imbalance before it can manifest or, if there is an imbalance, to correct it. The modern medical approach usually concentrates on the disease only after it has manifested. Modern science has in the past defined health as "absence of disease." According to Ayurveda, health is much more, a state of perfect balance of the physical and mental, leading toward immortality. Ayurveda is really *health*-oriented rather than *disease-oriented*.

It is the patient, however, who must establish perfect health by actively participating in the healing process. Ayurveda recognizes one's own Self as the ultimate healer, and the Ayurvedic physician becomes a partner with the patient to help the patient achieve perfect balance and develop an invincible immune system.*

The Ayurvedic preventive treatment *panchakarma*, is one of several types of Ayurvedic treatment designed to rejuvenate the physiology and the entire immune system. In addition to *panchakarma*, another treatment that is a popular part of Ayurveda is herbal food supplement. Ayurvedic herbal supplements are known for their rejuvenative and curative powers. These will be explained in Chapters Four and Five.

The goal of all Ayurvedic physical and herbal treatments is to remove imbalances from the physiology so that digestion and elimination work perfectly. This ensures (1) that impurities are not produced in the body by incomplete digestion; (2) that any unsuitable substances which contact the physiology through the environment are eliminated properly; and (3) that digestion can produce the highest possible quality of nutrients to support the body.

In a healthy body, the process of food digestion goes through various levels of refinement until the finest essential part of the food *(rasa)* is produced. This *rasa* created by the initial phases of digestion is then transferred with its nutrients to the lymphatic system and then to the blood, muscle, fat, bone, bone-marrow/nerve tissue, and then to the generative fluids, semen, and ovum. The very end product of the nutritional process is called *ojas*. *Ojas* is an ultra-refined substance known in Ayurveda as "vital essence." Such a substance is so far almost unknown to Western science. The *rasa* theory of Ayurveda describes the way in which nutritional material undergoes succeedingly finer states of transformation and separation into finer and more subtle nutrients until it reaches a final stage in human physiology as *ojas*, the ultimate nutrient.

According to Ayurveda, *ojas* is produced in humans in two different ways: in small amounts in a fully functioning digestive process; and in the practice of deep meditation, when subtle aspects of sound stimulate the physiology to produce *ojas*. It can take up to a month to produce *ojas* from food, but it is produced more quickly through meditation. In Ayurveda, *ojas* is synonymous with good health. (Ayurveda explains that health is latent in *ojas* as butter is latent in milk.) In some translations of the *Charaka Samhita, ojas* is likened to the Chinese theory of *chi'*. In degenerative diseases the *ojas* (or chi') does not circulate in the body but is excreted through the kidneys and bladder. A lack of *ojas* causes premature aging and degeneration of the immune system.

All of the restorative methods of Ayurveda are aimed at creating and conserving *ojas* and strengthening the entire immune system through the proper application of the *tridosha* theory. The *tridosha* theory of Ayurveda represents the main Ayurvedic method for diagnosis and treatment of the individual and is universally applicable for all people at all times.

*Ayurveda brings about a complete interconnection between all body parts, so that the physiology functions in a coherent manner. This coherence of bodily function will result in the natural restoration of an invincible immune system.

CHAPTER 4

THE
RASAYANA
TREATMENT

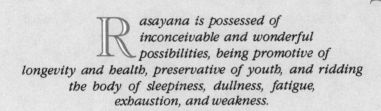

R asayana is possessed of
inconceivable and wonderful
possibilities, being promotive of
longevity and health, preservative of youth, and ridding
the body of sleepiness, dullness, fatigue,
exhaustion, and weakness.

Ashtanga Hridaya

Rasayana (rah-sigh-yah-na) is a comprehensive Sanskrit term* for procedures that rejuvenate the physiology, including the immune system. *Rasayana* or rejuvenation treatment is thus considered to be one of the most important of the eight separate branches of Ayurvedic science. The eight branches are as follows:

1. *Rasayana*	Rejuvenation treatment for regeneration of the immune system and entire physiology
2. *Kaya*	Internal or general medicine (diseases below the clavicle)
3. *Shalya*	Major surgery
4. *Shalakya*	Eye, ear, nose, throat, mouth (diseases above the clavicle)
5. *Bhuta vidya*	Psychiatry
6. *Bala vidya*	Pediatrics, obstetrics, gynecology
7. *Agada*	Toxicology
8. *Vajikarana*	Revitalization or fertility therapy

The *rasa* part of the word *rasayana* can be translated to mean taste, elixir, sap, serum, food juice, lymphatic fluid, plasma, essence, purified metal oxide, and even gravy or sauce. The *ayana* part of the word *rasayana* means "pathway", "to circulate" or "to have a home or abode." A *rasayana* treatment is a means of holistically restoring the immune system so that the bodily fluids circulate and find their home in perfect harmony in a balanced physiology, which in turn will create an invincible immune system. In times past the *rasayana* treatments were undertaken in a special facility, sometimes the physician's own home. A successful *rasayana* treatment radically rejuvenates the immune system. According to the ancient texts, some of the qualifications for a *rasayana* facility are that it be a place free from fear, that

---

* One of the many truly beautiful things about classical *Sanskrit*, which means elegantly polished or well put together, is the way in which approximately two hundred basic verb roots flower into thousands of verb stems, nouns, adjectives, and other parts of speech, so that the variety of creation can be expressed within a unity of language.

it be kept scrupulously clean, at all cost face away from a bitter wind, and have several inner and outer courtyards and gardens to provide visual beauty and protection from stress. Many exclusive health spas follow the prescriptions for a *rasayana* facility.

A traditional *rasayana* treatment requires about thirty days or one cycle of the moon. During this time several types of purification measures may be prescribed, such as an initial fast and some days of light diet. Usually, in order to cleanse the body of aggravated *doshas*, which tend to accumulate over time and cause imbalances, a series of physical measures are applied which are called *panchakarmas*, or the five basic actions. During this stage of the *rasayana* treatment, the body is cleansed and a nutritional evaluation is made that is appropriate for the patient's age and temperament, the season, and the climate.

Rasayana treatment can be generally divided into two main categories: (1) rejuvenation therapy *(panchakarma)* including nutritional correctional, and (2) food supplement therapy (herbal *rasayana*). Both types of treatments are gentle and effective and are usually combined into one complete program. Neither treatment has any side effects.

During the first stages of the *rasayana* program, the Ayurvedist determines the exact nature of the *panchakarma* treatment. *Rasayana* treatment is not considered suitable for the very aged, the very young (under seven years), the very infirm, those in some acute stages of disease, or for pregnant women.

Basic *rasayana* treatment may consist of minimal fasting, dietary correction and the application of appropriate five-action *(panchakarma)* therapy, including several types of mild internal cleansing. After the cleansing, the herbal *rasayana* treatment begins with herbal supplements appropriate to the constitutional type. These supplements may be taken within a normal daily routine at home, as recommended by the Ayurvedist.

For some Ayurvedists, the restoration of dietary principles in harmony with the *tridosha* represents from 50 to 100 percent of the treatment. However, accumulations of the *doshas* can be reduced best by the rejuvenation therapies of the *panchakaima* treatment.

The five basic physical treatments were revealed by the Vedic seers as corresponding to natural bodily cleansing functions that have become disturbed through dietary, emotional, or environmental stress. The purpose of *rasayana* is to cleanse the body so that it may again function in a more balanced and efficient manner. The treatments are simple and may be carried out rather easily, but since there are specific counterindications for the use of each, it is recommended that they only be prescribed or administered by a trained Ayurvedist.

The five basic actions
(panchakarma) are:

1. *Vamana*	Emetic treatment for balancing accumulated *kapha dosha*
2. *Virechana*	Purgation treatment for cleaning accumulated *pitta dosha*
3. *Basti Vijanyi*	Medicated or nutrient internal cleansing for accumulated *vata dosha* in the colon region
4. *Basti Sneha*	Lubricated internal cleansing for accumulated *vata dosha* in the colon region
5. *Nasya*	Nasal and ear cleansing for accumulated *kapha dosha* in the head and throat region

In addition to those primary therapies, *panchakarma* includes other therapies, such as Ayurvedic massage *(abhyanga)*, a very complete massage utilizing herbalized oils specific to each constitutional type. Specialized heat treatments of herbalized oil and herbalized steam *(swedana)* may also be used.

Other secondary therapies can be applied at each of several stages of the *rasayana* treatment, such as hydration and drying therapies, or heat and cooling therapies (including those of sunbathing or moonbathing). Many of these therapies have fallen out of fashion today because they are labor-intensive, expensive, and require exceptional service from a health care provider. However, with some study they can be easily mastered by health professionals and, with guidance and education, some may even be employed by patients themselves in a preventative health routine.

Rasayana treatments should be undertaken at the change of seasons for optimal benefit. The traditional *rasayana* treatment is completed in thirty days or less. During that time the diet and daily routine are watched carefully. For example, one eats in a quiet place and the food is eaten slowly enough to avoid stress. Leftover foods are to be avoided. After the *rasayana* treatment, the *doshas* will stay balanced for a time if given the opportunity. Herbal *rasayanas* may be recommended to insure the continued balance of the *doshas*.

An important part of the *rasayana* treatment is patient education. The self-help education provides maximum benefit during post-treatment periods. Ayurveda recommends preventative measures including dietetic instructions, exercise, and daily and seasonal routines. Chapter Seven describes the preventive Ayurvedic routine in detail.

At this point we would like to relate some of our personal experiences of Ayurvedic treatments. In the course of researching Ayurveda, we had been treated by several Indian Ayurvedic physicians *(Vaidyas)*. Pleased with the results of these *rasayana* treatments, we decided to try an extensive program recently made available in the United States.

For our research we chose the Maharishi Ayurvedic Medical Center™ at Fairfield, Iowa. The facility is a converted country estate with the colonnaded front porch of a Southern mansion. The building is surrounded by farmland and trees. Both of us visited the center for an initial evaluation of our basic constitutional type *(prakriti)* and a prescription of treatments to balance whatever *doshas* were accumulated in our bodies. Both of us followed a cleansing treatment at home for four days, then attended an orientation meeting and embarked on the *rasayana* treatment at the medical center.

LINDA'S TREATMENT DIARY

Initial Evaluation
I meet with Christopher Clark, M.D. for my preliminary evaluation. He says my primary constitutional type is *kapha,* with *pitta* as a secondary influence. He says *kapha dosha* is aggravated in my physiology and suggests friction or dry massage *(udhvarnta* massage) every day for the duration of my treatment. I am concerned about the friction on my skin so we compromise on dry massage every other day, alternating with medicated oil massage *(abhyanga)*. He also schedules me for Vedic herbal steam treatment *(swedana)*, and head massage with heated oil *(shirodara)*, a special Ayurvedic treatment. I am also scheduled for *pizichilli* treatment, which consists of heated oil poured in copious amounts over the body and gently massaged into the skin.

Home Preparation
Before I begin treatment of the clinic I take a course of herbs and nutrients recommended to loosen up the accumulated *doshas* and begin to cleanse the body. This is designed to maximize the purifying effects of the treatment.

Day Two of Treatment
This is my second day of *shirodara* treatment. Warm, herbalized oil is systematically dripped and poured over my forehead. I decide that *shirodara* is the most exquisite physical sensation available on the planet today, especially for professionals who do lot of mental work. During *shirodara,* the technician's hands do not touch my head. The falling droplets of warm sesame oil feel as if they are gently massaging the *inside* of my brain and give an incredible sense of relaxation.

Day Three of Treatment
The *shirodara* has eliminated a lot of my brain fatigue. I have some headache sensations but, as I am resting after treatment, almost imperceptibly the

headache dissolves into tears. I realize I have released some grief about my father's recent passing that I didn't know I had repressed. It is a great relief. I feel both lighter and stronger.

Day Four of Treatment
Pizza-chili time *(pizichilli).* Large amounts of warm oil are systematically poured over me and gently massaged in. It's a warming, balancing treatment for the *pitta dosha*. It has the effect of reducing my hunger. I am looking and feeling well. Funny, I have decreased at least one shoe size due to weight loss—my bedroom slippers have become too large!

Day Five of Treatment
Final evaluation. I look and act five years younger. My complexion is translucent and my eyes are bright. I have lost over five pounds without dieting or suffering.

SCOTT'S TREATMENT DIARY

Initial Evaluation
Today I met with Dr. Christopher Clark. Dr. Chris gave me a physical evaluation and determined my physiological type as *kapha* with *pitta* secondary. He suggested a treatment program especially for my body type, including medicated steam and oil therapy. I asked him how much rejuvenation I could expect and was told that after treatments most patients experience a loss of several years of biological age. Part of the initial evaluation is a routine physical exam, which includes blood pressure and other standard clinical tests.

Day One of Treatment
Today I was treated by two technicians who were very gentle and gave me a head massage with warm herbalized sesame oil. They told me that they would help to move the accumulated *doshas* and restore a more natural balance. After this I received a vigorous full-body massage with oil and herb powders that was very refreshing. Next came the *shirodara* treatment with warm herbalized oil on the forehead. This was an incredible feeling and very soothing. I wished that it could go on longer. After a shower and rest period, the technicians brought in some herbalized nose drops and began the nasal treatment *(nasya).* The drops smelled good and I am blowing my nose considerably after the treatment. It seems my vision has cleared and I notice a definite increase in my mental alertness and clarity of mind.

Day Two of Treatment
Today, after the full-body massage, the technicians took me to another room for the full-body medicated steam treatment *(swedana).* The technicians are

always so gentle and polite that it makes the program very pleasant. The steam is warm and I almost fall asleep. After a while they help to towel off the excess water and I take a shower. Today I am feeling more energetic after the treatment.

Day Three of Treatment
This morning I am looking forward to the treatment routine. Even though the whole routine takes about two hours, I'm thinking that I could be talked into doing this every day. After another head massage I got the *pizichilli* treatment. It is very relaxing, like passively swimming in oil. I wanted this to go on for at least another hour. Afterwards I took a shower and rested. On the way out I'm feeling more relaxed and stress-free than ever before. Linda tells me I look ten years younger.

Final Evaluation
I certainly feel younger. I'm writing on the evaluation sheet the benefits I have already experienced, which include better sleep, decreased hunger, no more indigestion, and reduced blood pressure. I look a lot younger, according to my friends and acquaintances.

Does all of this mean that Ayurveda is the secret to immortality? In our opinion, we feel that Ayurveda may be an important key in immortality research. Careful investigation of Ayurveda may point us in the direction of gaining that immortality which has long been sought by thoughtful persons in all times and cultures.

CHAPTER 5
HERBAL RASAYANAS

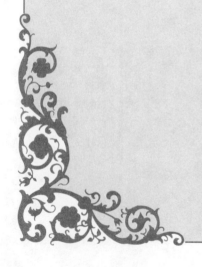

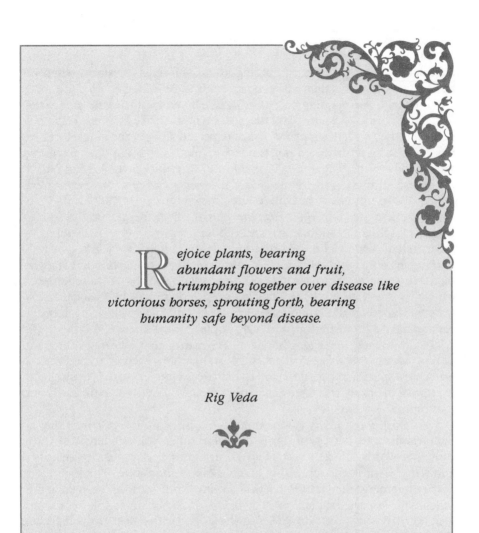

Rejoice plants, bearing
abundant flowers and fruit,
triumphing together over disease like
victorious horses, sprouting forth, bearing
humanity safe beyond disease.

Rig Veda

Jivaka, whose name means "one who gives life," was a student of Atreya, a great Ayurvedic scholar in the time of Buddha. Jivaka had almost completed his seven years of training as an Ayurvedic physician when his teacher gave him this final assignment. He was instructed to go eight miles into the jungle surrounding the city of Takashila. Within that perimeter, Atreya told him to bring back any plant that had no medicinal use. While other students returned with many plants, Jivaka remained alone in the jungle for three days. At last he returned empty handed, saying he could find no plant that did not have a medicinal use. Then Atreya pronounced that he had passed his course and was now free to set up his own practice of *rasayana* treatments. Jivaka ultimately became court physician to Lord Buddha.

There are over 5000 *rasayna* herbal supplements currently being manufactured and sold in India, and thousands more are manufactured by independent rural practitioners who grow herbs in their own gardens or gather them from the wild. Almost all of these preparations contain herbal ingredients in some form. An awareness of the special effects of these herbs or fruits may lengthen our lives. They are prepared as medicinal wines, decoctions, and medicinal oils and ghees for use internally as well as for massage, ear and nasal administration, and scalp application. There are also medicinal confections made with sugar, honey, and ghee in specified proportions, and others available as pills, powders, snuff and gargles. Each of these preparations has a specific action designed to remove congested *doshas* from specific areas of the body and to cleanse, strengthen, and rejuvenate the body and the immune system.

During the *rasayana* treatment, not only are the habits of the patient restructured, but a cleansing of mental attitudes is also undertaken. Those thoughts, words, and actions that are contributing to ill health are identified and the patient is encouraged to avoid them in the future. The Ayurvedist may recommend meditation that will automatically cleanse the mental attitudes. The Vedic texts specify that arrogant, disrespectful people should not take herbal *rasayana* treatments, nor should those that have not undergone the prescribed preparatory cleansing, nor those in whom there is a clear and definite indication of immediate death from a terminal illness.*

The aging process itself is considered to be a breakdown of the immune system that may respond to the *rasayana* treatment very well. Various recipes offer simple methods of relief from the stress of advancing age. These herbal *rasayanas* are designed to promote longevity and reduce or reverse

---

*Recently Maharishi Mahesh Yogi has announced the opening of a 1200-bed ultra-modern Ayurvedic Hospital in Maharishi Nagar, near Delhi, India. Intensive Ayurvedic treatment at this hospital is now offered for incurable or intractable diseases such as cancer, cardiovascular disease, multiple sclerosis, Alzheimer's syndrome and Parkinson's disease.

aging. *Charaka* says that there are two types of medicine: one promotes vigor in the healthy and the other destroys disease in the ailing. It is only a matter of degree, since the many herbal *rasayanas* do both jobs simultaneously. In the *Vedas,* the mylobalan fruits are cited as herbal supplements that serve as supreme vitalizers and restorers of youth. They are: *amla* fruit *(Embelica officinalis); harde* fruit *(Terminalia chebulia);* and *behada* fruit *(Terminalia belerica).*

The *mylobalan* fruits are all varieties of the Indian gooseberry. They are small, tart, gelatinous green fruits, similar in shape to the kiwi fruit. Each has a slightly different taste, and together they are used to compound the Ayurvedic panacea known as *triphalla (tri*—three, *phalam*—fruit). *Triphalla* is also a mild laxative, but its main use is as a restorative *rasayana.*

The mylobalan fruits are traditionally gathered by hand and many recipes are given for their employment as rejuvenators. All the mylobalan fruits are high in naturally occurring vitamin C and calcium. The *amla* fruit has the highest natural amount of vitamin C of almost any fruit or vegetable in the world, an average of .013 milligrams per gram. However, it is not the vitamin C content alone that makes it restorative, but its collection of different tastes *(rasa).*

The *harada* fruit contains five of the six tastes and its use, along with a cleansing diet, is a standard part of *rasayana* treatment. Ayurvedic literature states that the this fruit contains all of the six tastes except salt. The Tibetan texts say that it possesses all six tastes and has 17 of the 20 possible medicinal qualities. The 17 physiologically stimulating qualities are: soft, heavy, hot, unctuous, stable, cold, dull, excessively cold, smooth, liquid, dry, dense, light, clear/fragrant/sharp, dry, hard, fluid. Six different varieties of *harada* fruit are described, but only four are commercially used today. The most popular is called the *abhaya* and is known for its five-sectioned fruit. The *amla* fruit has its rejuvenating power in its cooling and tart quality. *Amla* means "sour" in Sanskrit. It is used as the basis of a traditional *rasayana* preparation named *chayavan prash.*

The following are some recipes and instructions for various traditional herbal *rasayanas* or food supplements, according to Ayurvedic texts. The procedures and recipes are only given to indicate the sophistication of the *rasayana* tradition. The practical application of these herbal *rasayanas* can be as simple as taking a natural food supplement daily.

SIMPLE *AMLA* VITALIZER

According to Ayurvedic lore, at the end of one year of stress-free living, on a full-moon day, after having fasted for three previous days, one should locate a grove of *amla* plants. One should gather the unspoiled ripe fruit in the hands and meditate on the fruits with eyes closed until they are transubstantiated by *Brahma* (creative intelligence) into ambrosia. (No time limit is specified for this action, but one assumes it occurs before sundown.) Dhanvantari (the ideal physician) instructs that when ambrosia dwells in these fruits, they become sweet as sugar and honey, unctuous, and soft. One may eat to fullness of these fruits, and by refraining from anger or passion may live far beyond the expectations of others.

THREE-MYLOBALAN VITALIZATION

This *rasayana* requires that a new, unseasoned cast iron pan be spread with the pulp of ripe *mylobalan* fruits and allowed to remain for a day and a half in the pan to oxidize. The paste is then collected by deglazing the pan with honey-water and the solution swallowed. After this has been digested, a meal of unctuous substances such as sesame oil, ghee, and honey should be eaten. After a year of regularly using this *rasayana* (which does not require a retired mode of life), the literature says one may live to a hundred years or more.

Harada, the chebulic *mylobalan,* is a great rejuvenator. Unlike *amla* and *behada,*, which are cooling in action, *harada* is a warming herb. In India it is called "the mother" because of its warm, nurturing action, and it is always given to those suffering from grief, especially to young children who have lost their biological mother. By tradition it is not given to pregnant women, to alcoholics, to those who have recently given blood or been weakened in any way, nor to those in the acute stages of a fever.

The potency of both *amla* and *harada* is gauged by the practitioner. Where a cooling action is required, *amla* is used; where a warming or heating action is required, *harada* is used. Where both actions are required together, the fruits are mixed. For *triphalla,* all three are combined into a fine powder *(churna)* and mixed with clarified butter (if a lubricating/heating action is desired) or mixed honey (if a lightening, astringent action is desired).

CHAYAVAN PRASH RASAYANA

Of all the *rasayana* preparations, the best known and most widely used in India is *chayavan prash*, a jam-like confection used more or less routinely for the nutritional maintenance of children, adults under stress, and the middle-aged. It is prepared from a recipe approximately 3000 to 5000 years old.

Chayavan, for whom the confection is named, was a great Vedic saint. The daughter of an Emperor prevailed upon him to relinquish his celibacy and serve as her husband. The saint prepared himself for marriage by taking *chayavan prash*. Even though *Chayavan* was extremely advanced in age, he became young and virile, with a well-knit body.

Although this recipe is several thousand years old, *chayavan prash rasayana* is still prepared today. In making *chayavan prash,* 500 ripe and unblemished *amla* fruits are used. (Cultivated fruits weigh about one ounce.) The gathered *mylobalan* fruits are washed and set aside. Four tolas (one tola equals approximately 10 grams) each of 34 additional herbs are combined with the fruits and tied loosely in a piece of cloth. They are then simmered in a copper vessel over a mild fire in 32 kilos of hot water until the mixture is reduced to 5 kilos. The herbal decoction is strained and the seeds of the mylobalan fruits are discarded. Then the remaining part of the mixture is fried in a combination of sesame oil and *ghee*. (Oil is known to be able to transport the medicinal powers of herbs, fruits, and flowers.) The fried mixture is then ground to a paste and mixed with the herbs and raw molasses. Then four additional herbs are added. The contents are stirred and reheated. When all cooking is finished, pure raw honey is added equal to half the quantity of the oil and *ghee*. The *Charaka Samhita* expressly forbids the heating of honey, since toxins may be formed. The sugar content of *chayavan prash* should be no more than 20 percent. Commercially made products often contain 50 percent sugar. Dosage is 1–2 teaspoons with warm milk morning and evening. One should take this *rasayana* for a minimum of six months to one year. In India, *chayavan prash* wrapped in sterling silver foil is served as a special after-dinner digestive.

Often *chayavan prash* is mixed with gold, silver, pearl, or other medicinally prepared metallic substances. Saffron, sandalwood, and musk are also used to improve the potency of this *rasayana*. During the *rasayana* treatment with *chayavan prash*, very acidic foods—or extremely spicy, sour, and pickled foods—are prohibited. The clarified butter used in the preparation acts as a natural preservative, so that *chayavan prash* retains its effectiveness for several years after manufacture.

Chayavan prash fulfills the requirement for an ideal medicine that is also a palatable food. It can be used by people of all ages with no side effects and with excellent results. It is also known to increase the vitality of couples who take it together with other appropriate food items. After a year of continuous use of at least 1 tablespoon per day, the *chayavan prash rasayana* will give a truly marvelous strength to the immune system, keeping the body free from colds and flu throughout the winter and give increased stamina and vitality in other seasons. It is an excellent *rasayana* for strengthening the immune system in general.

TRIPHALLA RASAYANA

Often *triphalla rasayana,* a combination of all three *mylobalan* fruits, is given to adolescents to help allay the stress of the period of adolescence. It is usually mixed with licorice, earth-mined salt, ginger, iron, gold, or silver and administered with other elements to increase its efficiency *(anupana)* that depend upon the specific effect desired. The traditional *anupanas* or vehicles for administration of medicine are water (usually warm, but occasionally cold), milk, *ghee,* butter or honey. It is advised that *ghee* and honey never be taken in equal amounts, since such a fifty/fifty combination is toxic. The dosage of this *rasayana* is up to 2 or 3 teaspoons per day for a period of one year, with *ghee* or honey and an appropriate diet.

One of the most common, popular, and useful herbs in Ayurvedic pharmacology is *brahmi.* An ancient Sinhalese proverb states, "Two leaves a day will keep old age away." The leaves of the *brahmi* plant resemble the two hemispheres of the human brain. *Brahmi* is cited as an effective aid for developing memory and intelligence. In India it is used to treat nervous disorders and mental retardation.

Brahmi calms the mind and relieves symptoms of mental stress. In Sanskrit it is named after the faculty of consciousness *brahma,* the creative factor. According to Ayurveda, *brahmi* unifies the functioning of the two hemispheres of the brain.

An interesting ambiguity arises in investigating the use of *brahmi* as a herbal tonic. There are over 120 different herbs described s similar to *brahmi.* Two separate and distinct herbs are described as *Brahmi* in the *Sushruta Samhita.* The first is known as "urban Brahmi" or "another Brahmi" *(mandukaparni)* and is in widespread commercial use in India today. (It is also called *Centella asiaticia-urban.*) It is a slender creeping plant especially abundant in the swampy areas of India and Shri Lanka and in the tropical regions of the Western Hemisphere. *Centella* is a favorite food of elephants, and their longevity is partly attributed to it. It is interesting that elephants are famed for good memory, and *brahmi* may be the reason for this legend. *Centella* is also called the Indian pennywort or Asiatic hydrocotyle.

In the Kerala region of South India, where the most conservative Ayurvedic medicine is practiced, another type of *brahmi* is used. When specified by pharmacies elsewhere it is called *Herpestis monneria.* The action of both *rasayana* drugs seems to be similar, and the potency of both may be increased by the use of special methods of preparation and administration.

Brahmi is said to be especially valuable for students, as it remedies following conditions: weak memory, forgetfulness, mental debility due to developmetal causes, and anxiety and stress during examinations. It is also used as a brain tonic for professionals who must do a lot of mental work, for the elderly who suffer memory loss, and as a general nerve tonic. *Brahmi* is also in popular use in India as an oil massage for scalp and hair treatment to prevent baldness brought on by an overheated condition of the head.

BRAHMI RASAYANA

After completing the necessary purification treatments, one who desires to undertake a *rasayana* treatment of *brahmi (herpestis monneria)* retires into a special room and recites the proper mantra (purposeful resonance) over a single dose of the expressed juice of the *brahmi* plant. In the evening, after the medicine has been digested, one takes a small portion of cereal without salt, adding boiled milk if desired. Using this for even a week improves memory, leads to an expansion of consciousness, and gives a glow to the complexion. It is said that after three weeks of correct and continuous *brahmi rasayana* treatment, *Saraswati* (the impulse of absolute knowledge) will strengthen the memory and the intellect will become much clearer and stronger.

BRAHMI RASAYANA
(in clarified butter)

Two measures of *brahmi* juice is combined with one measure of clarified butter, the *mylobalan* fruits and other herbs, then cooked. Medicated clarified butter is cooked in three stages: mild for oral indigestion; medium for massage or topical application; and well-done for use in a medicated suppository. This should be taken in a dose of 1 tola (10 grams), and followed after digestion by a meal of boiled rice, milk, and clarified butter. A complete *rasayana* of this elixir is said to be able to cure even heavy afflictions of epilepsy and insanity, and to cure the effects of poisons, as well as diseases of the skin.

BRAHMI RASAYANA
(in pill form)

The use of *Brahmi* in pill form allows more varied ingredients to be added to the basic formula, should the Ayurvedist desire. To make *brahmi* pills, the dried *brahmi* leaf is stewed in a copper pot for several days. The resulting *brahmi* paste is hand-rolled into small pills of approximately 25–50 milligrams each. Some very expensive *brahmi* pills are combined with gold and silver as well.

Brahmi pills are shade-dried or dried in the light of the full-moon. They are usually taken with clarified butter and milk. The combining of the herbs, copper, cooking process, and moonlight creates a synergistic effect. Any one alone would be useful, but together they achieve a holistic effect. *Brahmi* gently reorganizes the metabolism of the brain so that it runs more efficiently on its current blood supply, and more energy is freed for creativity and intellectual activity.

SOMA RASAYANA

In the early Vedic period, *Brahma,* the first Ayurvedist, is said to have created the *soma rasayana* for the prevention of death and decay of the physical body. The creeper described as the *soma* plant has 27 different species classified according to habitat, structure and potency. Procedures for administering the *soma rasayana* are described in detail in the *Rig Veda.* The preparation and administration of the *soma* ceremony given in the Ninth Mandala is the same as that described for the *soma rasayana* treatment, except that the fruits of *soma* shrubs and creepers that "trail upon the ground" should be ingested whole, rather than through drinking the plant juice.

To undertake *soma rasayana* treatment requires the use of a spa-like retreat for a period of thirty days. The treatment begins on a favorable day after the proper cleansing therapies. A whole plant is collected just as was advised for the *soma* ceremony. The bulb of the legendary *soma* plant, which is said to smell like clarified butter, is pricked with a golden needle and its milk collected in a golden cup. The Vedic texts strictly warn that no part of this *rasayana* should be undertaken without the proper protection of the required Vedic procedures. The participant drinks one swallow of the *soma* juice without tasting it, and then washes the mouth with water.

The *soma rasayana* is the most extreme of the purifying measures. What follows in the thirty days of the *rasayana* treatment is nothing less than a physical destruction of the body with a preponderance of inert material *(tamas)*, and its reconstruction with a rejuvenated physiology in which refined material *(sattva)* predominates. During the treatment one is not allowed the use of a mirror, since the bio-physical changes taking place are truly extreme. All passions, especially anger, must be avoided for an additional ten days following the completion of the treatment.

In the *Vedas* the *soma* plant is called the lord of medicinal herbs, and described as having fifteen leaves, gaining one leaf a day to the full moon, and shedding one leaf a day to the new moon. It is recorded that the *soma* plant has the ability to render itself invisible to a negative person. A successful completion of the *soma rasayana* treatment allows one almost unlimited strength and longevity. Dr. K.L. Bhishagratna stated in his translation of the *Sushruta Samhita* that successful completion of the *soma rasayana* allows one the (Christ-like) ability to ascend to heaven in one's own physical body. Many Ayurvedists lament that as far as our modern knowledge goes this *soma rasayana* is not currently within our reach. However, it may not be long before serious investigation of the *soma rasayana* can be reinstituted as part of our present-day immortality research on Ayurvedic life-extension techniques.

The herbal *rasayanas* described here represent only a sample of the most commonly used *rasayanas*. There are literally hundreds available. The unique quality of Ayurveda herbal *rasayanas* is that they are completely natural and positive in their effect. Ayurvedic *rasayanas* have none of the side effects associated with Western drugs. They are balanced within themselves and only serve to balance the patient.

The making of Ayurvedic herbal *rasayanas* is a pharmacological science in itself. Sometimes there are up to sixty different ingredients in a single preparation. Thousands of years in clinical applications have refined Ayurvedic *rasayanas*. Thus they help to fulfill the goal of Ayurveda to maintain or create a perfectly balanced physiology in the individual.

CHAPTER 6

RASASHASTRA: THE SCIENCE OF MINERAL REJUVENATORS

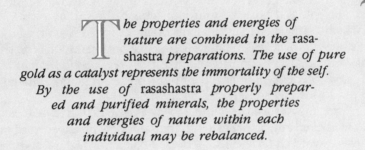

The properties and energies of nature are combined in the rasashastra preparations. The use of pure gold as a catalyst represents the immortality of the self. By the use of rasashastra properly prepared and purified minerals, the properties and energies of nature within each individual may be rebalanced.

Jnana Sunkalini Tantra

Rasashastra is the Ayurvedic discipline that is specifically concerned with the preparation of medicines from inorganic materials such as metals and minerals. *Rasashastra* outlines sophisticated procedures for unfolding the latent medicinal values of minerals so as to enhance their therapeutic action.*

Though it began in South India about 500 B.C., and reached a pinnacle around A.D. 1100, the main texts on *rasabastra* are attributed to Sidha Nagarjuna, a saint residing in India around the eleventh century.

According to Dr. V.B. Dash, a remarkable scholar of Indian and Tibetan medicine, a great debt is owed to the conservative abilities of the Tibetan medical scholars for preserving the Ayurvedic manuscripts that describe the various processes of *rasashastra*, including the actual processes of manufacture and administration. These descriptions are no longer available in the original Sanskrit, and must be retraced through the manuscripts found in Tibet. Whether Tibetan or Sanskrit in its original form, this Ayurvedic knowledge is still *sruti,* or revealed knowledge, since both traditions cite its originator as *Brahma*. The Buddhists add that it was revealed to Brahma by *rishi* Keshyapa, who cognized it as part of a discourse on immortality given by Lord Shiva to his mate and consort Parvati.

Rasashastra survives in India today as a branch of Ayurveda known as *sidha* medicine, originating in South India but now practiced in all regions. The Sanskrit word *sidha* means "perfected being" or "saint," and the pure *rasashastra* preparations, when properly prepared and administered, are able to cure the most serious and intractable diseases, many formerly classified as incurable.

Many Ayurvedic texts cite the uses of metals as food and medicine and describe both their tastes and actions. Gold is described as having a sweet and agreeable taste, acting as a restorative and subduing all three *doshas*. It is also described as cooling, antidotal to poisons, and beneficial to eyesight. Silver is described as having an acid taste, as laxative and cooling in its potency, and subduing *pitta* and *vata*. Copper is said to be astringent in its taste and liquefying in its potency. Iron generates lightness, quenches undue thirst, and subdues *pitta* and *kapha dosha*. Zinc and lead are described as having a saline taste and acting as vermifuges, liqueficants, and corrosives. Pearls, coral, diamonds, and lapis lazuli are beneficial to sight and calming and cooling in their potency.

Metals specifically mentioned in the *rasashastra* texts are described as undergoing a preparatory process known as *shodhana,* or purification. This initial purification allows *rasashastra* medications to be used without ill effect. After purification, the *rasashastra* medicines are prepared in a complicated process that consists of succeeding steps of oxidation or pre-digestion.

* Maharishi's *World Plan for Perfect Health*, 1985.

It is this unique process of pre-digestion that makes the mineral preparations safe and extremely valuable as medicinal substances.

Perhaps because of the exactness required in execution, or because of its sophistication and even inherent danger, the art of *rasashastra* is known to only a handful of scholars in the West. In one sense this lack of knowledge is deplorable, since research and the intelligent use of these metallic preparations could free countless people from the miseries of chronic degenerative and catastrophic diseases without the side effects of many medicines currently in use. In another view, the elusive nature of this knowledge is totally understandable, since the rediscovery of Ayurveda is only beginning. In all the extant texts on *rasashastra* there are warnings that, without the proper knowledge and instruction, nothing of real value may be learned and no healing power generated. If no special transformation occurs, because of lack of complete knowledge, one is left with nothing more than a heap of toxic metals.

However, if one is fortunate and assiduous, as well as crafty, as was Sidha Nagarjuna, one may learn the art of Indian alchemy, or *iatrochemistry*. Many legends exist about the career of Nagarjuna, an exceptional scholar of many interests, as well as a philosopher, chemist, administrator of a university and famous exponent of Buddhism.

One of the foremost legends about Nagarjuna's career holds that, due to lack of financial support for his university he was forced to use his yogic knowledge and fly across the ocean to consult a saint who knew the art of ancient chemistry. Nagarjuna achieved the ability to fly in this case by using two leaves of a rare tree. Since no one had ever before dropped in from the heavens to visit, the saint demanded that Nagarjuna surrender what he thought was the only leaf in order to learn the art of *rasashastra*. Thus the saint hoped to ensure that Nagarjuna could never return to society and reveal the secret art of ancient chemistry. Nagarjuna learned the art of *rasashastra* from the saint, then produced the second leaf and flew back to his university. With the secret knowledge he was then able to support a large body of scholars and monks.

In India today, many large pharmaceutical companies still manufacture *rasashastra* drugs according to the traditional texts. As will be seen in the following descriptions, these preparations are exceedingly time-consuming and intricate, and their effects are subtle, pervasive, and powerful, affecting mind, body, and consciousness in unity without any unpleasant side effects. They are unlike anything experienced in modern Western pharmacology.

According to the *sidha* system of medicine, metals as well as other substances have the qualities of the five *mahabhutas* (the basic elements described in Ayurveda). Physiological changes may be effected by using purified metals to balance the *doshas*. The *Rasa Ratnakar*, a famous Ayurvedic text, explains:

Just as a person who has won victory over death, just so by the use of rasa *and* rasayana, *and of the rasahastra minerals, it is possible to cure all kinds of disease, and to enjoy a long life with all the pleasures, while still keeping a very strong body, and without any weakness of the vital forces therein.**

In this *sidha* system of medicine, metals and metallic preparations are classified according to predominance of the five elements, as follows:

Element	Metal
Earth	Gold
Water	Lead
Fire	Copper
Vayu	Iron
Akasha	Zinc

Before the perfecting of herbal and mineral preparations of medicine, the Ayurvedist who understood the uses of the *rasayana* treatment was considered an exceptional being. With the understanding of the virtues of the *rasashastra* treatments, the Ayurvedist was considered to have divine healing capacities.

A large number of different mineral preparations are commercially manufactured in India today. The specific methods of manufacture of these mineral remedies includes the complete oxidation of minerals into an exceedingly fine mineral ash, *(bhasma),* preparation of pulverized gemstones *(pishti)*—a process in which gemstones are minutely pulverized with milk or rosewater—and the laborious preparation of *makaradwaj,* a re-sublimed sulfide that is prepared with or without the use of gold as a catalyst, and the preparation of finely ground ashes of iron *(loha).*

BHASMA

The *bhasmas* are mineral medicines that first undergo a special preliminary purification process known as *shodhana.* This process consists of eight to eighteen separate operations that begin with the creating of metal foil one

* Regarding death: In the *Charaka Samhita* the author makes the subtle and fascinating discrimination that, although the diamond noose of death is *unbreakable,* through the proper use of *mantra* (purposeful resonance or words that have a known effect) and the proper use of Ayurvedic medicine, the unbreakable noose of death may be *dissolved.*

sesame seed in thickness. After the metal is pounded to "airy thinness," it is heated and drawn into a fine wire. The wire is heated red hot and then cooled in plant juices one or more times. Following this purification it is ready to be made into medicinal ashes of metal. Iron, tin, lead, gold, silver, copper, zinc, and other metals are powdered and reduced through heat to their oxides. They are then mixed with juices of herbs and pulverized in various liquids. Then they are mixed with ground herbs, powdered and incinerated 21–1000 times. The result of this process is a very fine oxidized powder of metal that cannot be reconstituted. It is called a *bhasma*.

PISHTI

Gemstones and soft mineral elements are prepared by the operation known as *pishti*. It is the creation of *bhasma* without the use of fire. The properties of *pishti* medicines are cooling, soothing, and strengthening. Pearl, mother-of-pearl, conch shell, coral, red jasper, and other minerals are powdered finely in a mortar and rubbed in milk or pure rosewater for 21–100 days. A very thin paste forms that is rolled by hand into very small pills, and dried in moonlight, sunlight, or shade, depending upon the effect desired. This soft mineral medicinal preparation is called *pishti*.

MAKARADWAJA

The secret process for making *makaradwaja*, or re-sublimed sulfides, is the ultimate achievement of *rasashastra**. Purified minerals (symbolic of the vital essence of Lord Shiva) are combined in a mortar with sulfur (symbolic of the vital essence of his consort Parvati) in a proportion of 1:2. The resulting black compound, called *kajali*, is heated in a fireproof bottle that is buried in sand for 72 hours. Every eight hours the heat is increased until, at the third day with the heat at its highest, a cork is applied to the neck of the bottle. The red sulfide collects at the neck of the bottle as the heat is reduced. If gold is used as a catalyst, the preparation is called *dwiguna makaradwaja*. If it is not, the preparation is called *rasa sindhur*. The preparations are used to treat different ailments, even though their chemical composition may seem the same.

This process of mixing sulfur with *makaradwaja* is repeated up to one hundred times for the highest potency, known as *shataguna* (one hundred, or even one thousand oxidations) *makaradwaja*. This is an expensive

---

* Thakkur. *The Pocketbook of Herbal Remedies.*

preparation, used mainly for the treatment of chronic degenerative and cata-strophic diseases, including senile debility and impotence. *Makaradwaja* is also used in cases where full *rasayana* treatment may not be carried out.

LOHA BHASMA

A medicinal preparation of completely oxidized iron is called *loha bhasma*. Many forms of inorganic iron are toxic and difficult to assimilate, but accord-ing to research conducted by leading Ayurvedic pharmacies in Indra, this com-pound is assimilated into the bloodstream very easily. To prepare *loha bhasma,* a piece of iron is soaked in a specific acid solution until it is oxidized. Then it is finely powdered and roasted with cow's milk or ghee, oil or herb juices. The roasting and powdering process is repeated from 21 to 100 times. *Mand-hur bhasma* (dross of molten iron) is made after twenty-one separate oper-ations.

SHILAJIT

Another mineral drug with an ancient history is the mineral pitch tonic of the Himalayas, known as *shilajit* and described in the section on medicine of the *Charaka Samhita*. There is some dispute as to whether this compound is the same as that now being commercially harvested in the mountains of Nepal and Singapore and used in the manufacture of both Ayurvedic and Chi-nese herbal medicines. In any case, the action of the two compounds seems similar enough to explore the usefulness of mineral pitch in both its present-day and historical contexts. *Shilajit* (destroyer of weakness) is the bituminous exudate of granite rocks, a sort of "blood of the rock" secreted during the hot summer months. It is scraped off the rocks and purified either by sun-shine or by heating. *Charaka* described seven different types of mineral pitch, the four most common being gold, silver, copper, and iron. Of these, the *shilajit* from iron is considered the most beneficial.

Mineral pitch is either extracted or used in conjunction with other mineral or herbal preparations. In a traditional *rasayana, shilajit* is taken in conjunction with milk. The traditional dose is from 1 to 4 tolas (10–40 grams) for a minimum of one week, a medium of three weeks, and a maximum of seven weeks. Because it is thought to be the "essence of sunshine" and to balance all three *doshas* at one time, *Charaka* states that, when properly pre-pared and administered, *there is no curable disease on earth that mineral pitch cannot cure.* During the *shilajit rasayana* no legumes are permitted in the diet, since they are thought to interfere with its curative properties.

Special combination preparations of mineral, plant and herbal drugs are used for severe illness, diseases of aging, and certain types of sexual dis-function. When they are used as revitalizers or *ojas*-producing supplements, these applications come under the branch of Ayurvedic medicine called *Vajikarana*, revitalization treatment.

In Ayurveda revitalizers are used as preventives to awaken, strengthen, and conserve procreative muscles and energies so they remain healthy for an entire lifetime. These compounds are also used to harmonize the masculine and feminine energies in partners so that they attain maximum appreciation and harmony, avoid sterility and infertility, and prevent divorce due to emotional or sexual dissatisfaction.

Each constitutional type may require a different type of revitalization treatment. The *vata* type is often treated with the seven mineral ashes (copper, iron, tin, silver, gold, lead, and zinc), plus a non-toxic purified form of *Nux vomica* herb. The *kapha* type is known for an innate sexual capacity, and may only be treated with *shilajit* and unctuous food. The *pitta* type often requires cooling and soothing herbs and treatment with pearl *bhasma*.

VASANT KUSAMAKAR RAS

This preparation is used for virility and for serious conditions such as asthma, diabetes, aging, and impotence. The mineral elements are potentized and then ground in plant juices and milk for an extended period of time, through seven different heating and cooling operations. It is then taken with milk, butter or honey for 30–90 days.

NAVA RATNA
(nine gems)

The renowned nine-gems preparation is rarely seen today in even the most prestigious pharmaceutical houses of India. It is costly and extremely time-consuming to make, requiring a minimum of one thousand separate operations and two years' preparation time. The only preparation that requires more time is *abhrak bhasma* (oxidized mica), which requires a minimum of five years *daily* preparation. To make the nine-gem medication, nine different gemstone powders are pulverized in the juice of sandalwood and rosewater at least 1000 times and then combined in equal proportions. One formula for the *nava ratna* preparation is as follows: *

---

* It may not be too long before Makaradwaja and other exceptional rasashastra preparations will be recognized as a unique and extremely powerful means of achieving infinite life-extension on an individual basis.

Heera pishti	Diamond
Panna pishti	Emerald
Yakut pishti	Ruby
Neelmani pishti	Sapphire
Mukta pishti	Pearl
Praval pishti	Red Coral
Sange Yashm pishti	Jasper
Trikantmani pishti	Amber
Hingula pishti	Cinnabar

The treated gemstones *(pishti)* are sometimes combined with musk, saffron, mica and *makaradwaja*. Very tiny pills of approximately $\frac{1}{32}$ of a grain are prepared. One pill a day is taken on an empty stomach with warm or tepid water for thirty days, usually starting with the full moon. For those fortunate enough to obtain it from an authentic source, the nine-gem *rasayana* may be the Ayurvedic treatment of choice for catastrophic illness, since it is known to be kind to the patient and merciless to the disease. This compound is also famous for its subtle ability to refine the physiology of healthy persons.

The art and science of Ayurvedic pharmacy is very highly developed. We now have the technology available to make the traditional manufacture of these preparations almost effortless and reduce the time required to months rather than years for even the most complicated products. Since all Ayurvedic medicines are prepared to have no side effects whatsoever, research leading to the judicious introduction of these compounds into a more general use will be of inestimable value to humankind.

CHAPTER 7

AYURVEDA
AND
THE LIFE CYCLE

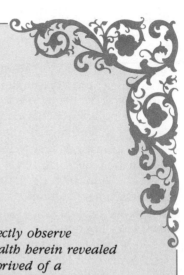

*Those who correctly observe
the rules of health herein revealed
will not be deprived of a
hundred years of healthy life.*

Charaka Samhita

Thousands of years ago Atreya, the great Ayurvedist, revealed the knowledge that the individual is nothing more nor less than a microcosm of the entire universe. All things present in the universe are present in the individual. Both have cycles of life; both have a source (the mind of God), and existence, and a dissolution. Realizing this magnificent unity of each individual with the universe is an important step on the path of wellness. Harmonizing individual behavior with the universal cycles of nature allows one to move through life with the greatest freedom, happiness and serenity.

The many natural cycles continually move, one within the other, ranging from the longest expansion and contraction cycle of the entire universe, a cycle of billions of years, to the vibratory cycles of the minutest atomic particles, which have a duration of only billionths of a second. Because everything we do or experience is part of the unity of nature, we humans experience these cycles continuously.

Ayurveda works very well as a preventive health modality because it recognizes that life is a dynamic condition that must be maintained in balance by intelligent action through daily, monthly, and seasonal cycles. This emphasis on continuous self-care allows us to cultivate longevity and maximum vitality throughout the entire life cycle. Using Ayurvedic knowledge to bring the physiology into balance (balancing the *doshas*), we are able to harmonize our personal and individual life cycles with the cycles of nature and thus live a truly natural life in complete health.

Even when we are in very good health, the working of the physiology causes *doshas* to accumulate in the body. This accumulation is the prerequisite for the manifestation of any and all diseases. If the body is in balance illness will not occur, no matter how strenuous the demands made upon it. The simple preventive methods of Ayurveda are designed to remove accumulated *doshas* from the body quickly and easily. The result of this continual cleansing is freedom from disease. As Ayurvedic wisdom is incorporated into the life style, the result will be continuous freedom from disease. Continuous freedom from disease will result in contentment, longevity, and ultimately in enlightenment.

The signs that the *doshas* are accumulating are simple and clear and so are the Ayurvedic methods for their counteraction and removal. *Vata dosha* is said to be the strongest of the *doshas*. It is the most subtle and elusive, and can cause the other *doshas* to move out of balance because of its strong "moving" quality. Control of *vata dosha* is therefore most important when attempting to maintain a preventive balance. The aggravation of *vata dosha* is said to be the causative factor in over 50 percent of all diseases.

When *vata dosha* is aggravated one may experience pain, nervousness, restlessness, dryness, cracking, roughness in sensitive areas of the body, and problems with the joints. Ayurvedic measures used to neutralize and expel *vata* are:

1. Oil application (a light golden sesame oil is best for most purposes)
2. Heat application (dry or moist heat depending upon the condition)
3. Pressure (such as massage or support bandage to the area of *vata* accumulation)

Oil, heat, and massage will always control vata dosha.

When *pitta dosha* is accumulated, the perceptible signs are fever, redness, heat, sourness of body and mind, indigestion, itching, anger, and irritation.

Ayurvedic measures used to neutralize and expel *pitta dosha* are:

1. Coolness (moonlight)
2. Coldness (cooling substances such as yogurt, pomegranate, lemon, buttermilk)
3. Wetness (bathing, wet compresses)
4. Air

(The vedic texts also advise the use of soothing elements such as sweet music, fragrant flowers, and the company of true friends.)

When *kapha dosha* is accumulated, the perceptible signs are swelling, blistering, mucus formation, dullness and sleepiness. Ayurvedic means to neutralize and expel *kapha dosha* are:

1. Friction (dry massage)
2. Exercise
3. Fasting or reduction of food
4. Reduction of sleep
5. The medicinal use of herbal inhalants

Using these simple Ayurvedic procedures routinely provides for continous and regular elimination of the *doshas* and helps to free the body to accomplish its many other tasks. The signposts that the lifecycle is progressing normally are: freedom from pain, a glowing complexion, bodily strength, desire to take nourishment, normal hunger, evacuation, restful and refreshing sleep with a calm awakening, and thorough elimination of all bodily waste. The result of these proper functions is contentment—satisfied mind, intellect, senses, and body. The result of this harmony is *ayus*, or life. *Ayus* maintained indefinitely through the use of Ayurvedic life cycle routines brings infinite life extension toward immortality.

DAILY ROUTINE

In order to maintain vitality, Ayurveda recommends regularity in daily, monthly, and seasonal routines. Best results are obtained by innocently incorporating these simple routines into normal activities. Some of these practices are considered old-fashioned and conservative, but they preserve and protect the physiology so that life may be lived at its highest potential.

The daily routine begins with the recommendation to rise early. This puts us in tune with the rhythm of nature (which begins a fresh cycle each morning.) Usually "early" means some time between 4:30 and 7 A.M., depending on the season. On arising, evacuate the bladder and the bowels. Clean the teeth, including gum massage with oil and herbal powders. Tongue scraping or brushing is recommended at this time to remove the toxins and waste material that have accumulated overnight. The hair and nails are considered waste products *(malas)*, so shaving if needed, and the trimming of nails and beard are considered part of the eliminative routine to be done at this time.

To control the ever-present accumulation of *vata dosha*, anoint the body with oil daily before bathing. A small amount of warm sesame oil may be gently massaged from head to toe. Sesame oil diminishes all three *doshas* and is appropriate for all body types. The oil is prepared by gentle heating. It can be made a quart or more in advance and then stored. The small amount used each day is then rewarmed before the massage.

According to Ayurveda, body massage begins by massaging the head vigorously and then putting a little oil in the ears and nose. The rest of the body is massaged, including the soles of the feet. The amount of oil used should be from an eighth to about a third of a cup. After 5 to 10 minutes the oil has absorbed the toxins eliminated through the skin during the night. (During the daily routine some of the oil is absorbed through the skin and nourishes the body tissues. No more than 1 teaspoon of the oil is actually absorbed into the skin—equal to approximately 60 calories.) After thirty days of regular oil massage the appetite is naturally reduced and the hair, skin, and nails are stronger and more attractive. When the daily massage is completed, take a shower or bath to wash off the excess oil and the bodily toxins. For morning joggers or before aerobic exercise or weight lifting, it is best to lubricate the body first, then exercise and shower.

Now it is time for morning meditation. Meditation is a primary Ayurvedic health routine, not to be missed, since it provides the basis for all the other healthful activities to take place. Meditation is followed by worship according to one's beliefs. When all these steps have been completed, it is time to dress for the day's activities.

These recommendations may seem lengthy, but when they become habitual they do not take much extra time. To get the best results, follow all of the recommended routine. However, if all of it cannot be done, then do

68

as much as can be done. Perhaps the full-body massage can only be done on weekends at first. It is best to begin the routine on a weekend to allow time to integrate the changes into the normal daily routine. The wonderful feelings of increased cleanliness, freshness, invigoration, and strength that follow the introduction of this routine will help to reinforce it as a daily habit.

Exercise taken after the morning meditation is also recommended. If it is not done in the morning, it should be done sometime during the day. The Ayurvedic attitude towards exercise is one of moderation and regularity. Since intake and expenditure of air *(vayu)* can aggravate many diseases, Ayurveda says it is healthful to exercise to half of one's normal capacity (that is until a mild perspiration forms on the forehead, or until forced to breathe through the mouth to get sufficient air.)

For example, a jogger may run 2 miles each day, three days a week; Ayurvedists would then advise to jog 1 mile per day. Or, if we have been doing a half hour of aerobics every other day we should ideally do 15 minutes every day. A *kapha* body type should do more exercise than a *vata* or *pitta* body type, since *kapha* tends toward inertia and requires more "moving" of the *kapha dosha* to maintain balance. Exercise is a matter of common sense and should never be overdone. It is good either to exercise before meals or to wait for an hour after meals.

Kapha constitutional types should avoid eating breakfast and fast with juice until at least 10 A.M. *Pitta* and *vata* constitutional types should have breakfast. Breakfast should be somewhat light and in accordance with one's body type and the season. After the morning routine comes work or other daily activity until lunch time. Ayurveda recommends that lunch be the main meal of the day and that it be balanced nutritionally according to body type. Cycles are determinants of longevity, so when the sun is highest in the sky the inner digestive fire called *agni* is also at its peak. Those with weak digestion should never eat heavily after sunset.

Ayurveda also makes the point that it is very important to focus on the food while eating (rather than to watch television or read a book.) Because taste is so important to the balance of the *doshas*, digestion functions better when attention is on the food. The eyes are mainly controlled by the functioning of *pitta*, so in the Ayurvedic sense, the eyes also "digest" what they see, and it is important to note the pleasant visual aspects of the meal. It is said that the digestive fire is responsible for the digestion and assimilation of our food. Therefore we must avoid too much liquid before or after meals, although small amounts aid in digestion. Ice water or any other very cold liquid are to be avoided, as they tend to put out the digestive fire and impair the process of digestion. A short rest, but not a nap, after lunch is recommended.

When the afternoon's activities are completed, the evening routine begins with meditation. Then comes the evening meal, which should be smaller, lighter, and easier to digest than lunch. Dinner is prepared to suit the individual constitutional type and the particular season of the year. It is suggested that a brief walk be taken after dinner and followed by some relaxing activities. A bath or shower right after eating would not be good for digestion, but immediately before a meal is all right.

There is an Ayurvedic routine for the evening and night, and at least 4000 years before Benjamin Franklin advised it in *Poor Richard's Almanac*, Ayurveda recommended early rising and early retiring for health, happiness and longevity. Proper sleep is very important for optimal health, and Ayurveda has some suggestions regarding the proper way to sleep. Of course, it is important to sleep in a quiet, comfortable place. Ayurveda recommends sleeping on the right side, if possible. Sleeping with the head facing East or South is advised. Sleeping in the day is not recommended, since this increases dullness *(kapha dosha)* and may create an imbalance. Sleeping right after eating may have a similar effect.

Please keep in mind the principles of diet discussed in Chapter Three. These simple Ayurvedic principles added to the daily routine will do a lot to keep the *doshas* in balance and greatly improve health and longevity.

MONTHLY ROUTINES

The lunar fertility cycle in women is the most obvious monthly cycle in human life. Ayurveda describes this cycle and other closely associated cycles dealing with motherhood and sexuality and offers many ways to preserve health during menstruation, ovulation, conception, pregnancy, and lactation.

When a couple is interested in conceiving a child they want to produce as healthy a child as possible. They may also have preference for a boy or a girl. According to Ayurveda, the first requirement for producing healthy children is healthy parents. This means parents should start to prepare themselves for parenthood several months in advance or sooner. The Ayurvedic routines strengthen the parents' physiology in preparation for having children. Ayurvedic therapies previously described are recommended. These include the *rasayana* treatment and a conscious restructuring of diet and life style. The *panchakarma* treatments and *rasayana* food supplements will increase the likelihood of healthy and happy offspring. *Panchakarma* rejuvenation treatments before pregnancy are important for older, first-time parents, or as a non-invasive addition to other fertility measures.

Ayurveda suggests the diet for prospective parents may include the addition of milk products, which generally have a positive effect on male virility. Men may improve fertility by the eating of milk products and other unctuous (oily) foods in moderation over several months. If appropriate, Ayurvedic herbal rejuvenators and other remedies may be used in preparation for conception.

Ayurveda notes that menstruation marks the beginning of the fertility cycle, not its conclusion. A normal menstrual cycle usually occurs during the waning half of the moon and takes just three days (about 72 hours) to complete. If pregnancy is to be attempted during the next thirty days, Ayurveda advises complete rest during these three days of menstruation. Any activities that aggravate the *doshas* at this time will appear in the ovum at the time of next ovulation. The *panchakarma* treatments are not to be undertaken during the first three days of menstruation.

Excesses of any kind should be avoided when conception is desired. This includes too much eating, drinking or fasting, as well as unleashed fear, anger, or any other negative emotions. Moderation helps to prevent imbalances that could interfere with the conception. Drinking warm milk with almonds afterwards is an excellent rejuvenator and helps to replace bodily fluids for both partners.

According to Ayurveda, conception during the even days of the monthly fertility cycle (counted from the first day of menstruation) tends to produce a male child and conception during the odd days of the cycle tends to produce a female child. The best days for conceiving a healthy son are days 4, 6, 8, and 12 of the menstrual cycle. The best times for conceiving a healthy daughter are days 5, 9, and 11.

The twilight periods between dark and light are considered inappropriate times for conception. Dawn and dusk are juncture points, *(sandhi)* and it is advised to rest or meditate during these transition times. There are various Ayurvedic medicinal preparations that can help to maintain a balanced and healthy pregnancy.

According to the *Charaka Samhita*, "The child tends to resemble those things which the mother thinks in her mind during conception." Ayurveda explains that the fetus begins to form during the conception period, which is why it should be a time of happiness and health. Five factors are responsible for the successful outcome of pregnancy: the health of the mother, the health of the father, the wholesomeness of the routine during pregnancy, the consciousness of the child, and the quality of the nutrients produced by the mother.

The pregnant woman is to be kept happy, relaxed, and satisfied. As much as possible she should have all her desires fulfilled. This will help to provide a balanced and successful pregnancy. Sometimes a pregnant woman desires something unusual, such as special foods. Ayurveda explains that these desires are often those of the unborn child, and their satisfaction may fulfill a nutritional need of the fetus.

Ayurveda says that the heart of the mother is connected to the heart of the fetus through the channels that carry nutrients from her to the baby.

Good care and protection of the mother at this crucial time is essential to the good health of the child. Modern medicine is coming to the Ayurvedic conclusion that the well-being of the mother is the well-being of the unborn child.

Ayurveda recommends special attention to the mother's diet during pregnancy since this is also the diet of the fetus. No alcohol, tobacco, or other toxins should be ingested at this time and the mother's diet should be balanced according to the demands of the body type and season.

Ayurveda recommends that the following activities be *avoided* during pregnancy:

Sleeping habitually on the back
Constant grief
Thinking negatively about others
Stealing
Anger
Physical or verbal abuse (either giving or receiving)
Excessive sleeping
Sleeping in the open air and/or moving around alone at night
Addiction to wine, alcoholic beverages, drugs or other toxins
Eating a lot of pork
Eating too much fish
Too many sour foods
Too many sweet foods
Too much salt
Too many pungent or spicy foods
Too many bitter foods
Too many astringent foods
Too much thirst
Too much hunger
Seats that are uncomfortable or too high
Traveling on bumpy or rough roads
Undue stress, physical or mental
Unsuitable or excessive exercise
Foods that are too hot in temperature or too spicy
Suppression of natural urges, such as defecation or flatus
Frequent looking down deep wells, holes or places water falls
Exposure to unpleasant sounds

When a healthy pregnancy has been completed and the child is born, Ayurveda gives further hygienic and practical suggestions too numerous to explain here. Ayurveda is complete in its scope regarding the science of obstetrics, gynecology, and pediatrics, and there are many volumes available that describe these areas of study in detail.

Ayurveda describes the causes of twins and multiple births as being the quality and effect of the genetic material of the parents and the *doshas* dominant in the genetic material at conception. The *vata*-genic quality of modern fertility drugs that stimulate the mother's body to ovulate is considered by Ayurvedists to be so strong that it produces multiple ova, thus accounting for multiple births to such women.

When caring for the new-born child, Ayurveda recommmends breast-feeding, if the milk is of good quality. At the beginning of each feeding, the mother is advised to express and discard the first few drops of milk from each breast so that the child will receive only fresh milk.

SEASONAL ROUTINES

One of the major advantages of Ayurveda is that health is evaluated on an individual basis, and the evaluation is repeated regularly, especially at the junction point of the seasons. Ayurveda divides the yearly cycle into six seasons. For our purposes, we will deal with only three—spring, summer, and fall/winter.

Ayurveda says that diseases arise at the juncture point of the seasons. During the ten-day period before and after the change of seasons, the diet should be adjusted according to body type to harmonize with the cyclical changes. This is also the usual time to institute or adjust preventive health measures on a formal basis. Being aware of the cyclical changes puts us in tune with the natural law that governs our constantly changing environment and, indeed, the evolution of our own lives.

SPRING
(March–June)
Kapha Season

The accumulated winter snows begin to melt and flow. Cold weather gives way to warming winds and growing plants. This is analagous to the *kapha dosha*, which has accumulated and now needs to be eliminated. The body usually desires to do some spring cleaning. For *kapha* body types especially, this is a time to cut back on *kapha* foods and increase exercise. *Kapha* is aggravated in this season. Since *kapha* is cold and wet in action, many people get spring colds at this time, and are best served by a change of nutritional routine.

SUMMER/FALL
(June–October)
Pitta Season

During the summer the action of the sun influences our health and our lives. As the sun comes out and warms up the earth, *pitta dosha* tends to accumulate in our physiology and to reduce the *kapha dosha*. As we experience this heating and drying process, the body requires more relief from the heating action of *pitta*, and one is naturally attracted to cooling activities such as swimming. The effect of *pitta* may be counter-balanced by avoiding foods that are very salty, sour, or pungent, and hot in temperature. Sweet, heavier food may be favored, along with cool foods and drinks.

FALL/WINTER
(November–February)
Vata Season

The transition from summer to fall and winter requires the most vigilance in health care, since many diseases begin because of improper health habits at the onset of autumn. *Vata dosha* is personified in the rough, dry, northerly winds that begin in fall. Even during snowfall there is still dryness and coldness, which increases the rapid accumulation of *vata*. The diet should be enriched with dairy products and oily, higher calorie foods and warm liquids such as teas, soups and stews. Dry, light foods that aggravate *vata dosha* should be reduced in the diet. When the health is properly cared for during the fall/winter season, then the transition to the spring will be almost effortless, and another yearly cycle of health will be maintained.

LIFESPAN ROUTINES

The orderliness of natural law is expressed in the various cycles within cycles. The seasonal cycle functions within the yearly cycle and the yearly cycle unfolds into our life cycle. Ayurveda defines the "normal" lifespan of a human being as that period appropriate to the age in which he or she lives. Ayurveda divides these ages into periods of less and greater stress in the world. When a preponderance of individuals in a society are living a balanced, healthy life, the society as a whole reflects this. This principle of coherence points up the transformative power of Ayurveda for creating a stress-free world.

An individual who lives under stressful social conditions cannot expect to live as long as an individual who lives in a more stress-free society.

This makes sense because stress causes wear-and-tear on the physiology, which we see as aging. Stress, in a general sense, is the cause of disease and death.

The normal lifespan is defined in Ayurveda as at least 100 years. There are many references in Vedic literature to a normal individual lifespan of 1000 years, 10,000 years, 100,000 years, 1,000,000 and more. This is a much more interesting idea of "normal"!

Ayurveda divides a normal lifespan into four separate phases. Each phase requires different types of social obligations and activities. The first division of the lifespan is called *brahmacharya*, which can be understood as the *student period* of life from age 1 to 25. This is a period of physical and psychological development allied to education and increasing experience of life.

The second division, from age 25 to 50, is called *grihasta,* the householder or *family period* of life. Usually this time is reserved for marriage and creation of a family. Also, this is the time of concentration on establishing a career and making many social contacts.

The third division is called *vanasprastha,* a *semi-retirement period* that lasts from age 50 to 75. One's career and family have been established and the social duties may be somewhat lighter. There may be more time for activities that are relaxing and informative. Humanitarian and charitable acts may take precedence over a career at this stage.

The fourth and final division is called *sanyasi,* the *complete retirement period,* undertaken from age 75 to 100. The ideal at this stage of life is to complete the process of Self-realization or enlightenment if it has not been accomplished earlier in the life cycle.

The purpose of Ayurveda is to extend our normal life span beyond 100 years, including a lengthier period of active health through principles of preventive care. Ultimately Ayurveda directs us toward immortality. Although the unified field is always immortal and unchanging, the body, the *chhandas* aspect of our physiology, continually changes and can be preserved through Ayurveda, the ancient science of infinite life extension.

CHAPTER 8

A VISION OF THE
POSSIBILITIES FOR THE
INTEGRATION OF
AYURVEDIC MEDICINE INTO
THE MODERN PRACTICE OF
PREVENTIVE HEALTH CARE

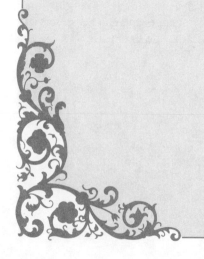

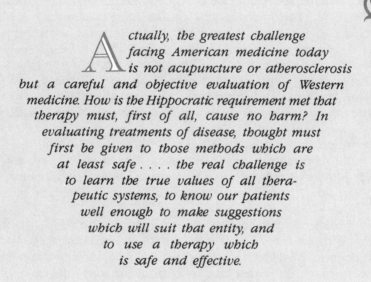

*A*ctually, the greatest challenge
facing American medicine today
is not acupuncture or atherosclerosis
but a careful and objective evaluation of Western
medicine. How is the Hippocratic requirement met that
therapy must, first of all, cause no harm? In
evaluating treatments of disease, thought must
first be given to those methods which are
at least safe . . . . the real challenge is
to learn the true values of all therapeutic systems, to know our patients
well enough to make suggestions
which will suit that entity, and
to use a therapy which
is safe and effective.

C. Norman Shealy, M.D.
The Pain Game

Less than two hundred years ago a theory of humoral pathology, which accounted for individual constitutional types and was not unlike aspects of the *tridosha* theory in some of its applications, was in common use in the United States for diagnosis and treatment of patients. Since that time allopathic medicine has come to emphasize germ theory in its practice. The individualizing effect of awareness of constitutional type has been largely ignored, and as a result a lack of wholeness is felt within all segments of our large and pluralistic community of health practitioners. In fact, the American Medical Association in 1976 made an ongoing commitment to restore holism and spirituality to the practice of medicine in our country.*

In all branches of modern medicine enormous amounts of scientific data are available. Yet health care costs continue to rise and the quality of care diminishes. The inadequacy of institutional medicine may be blamed in part on the lack of a unifying medical paradigm that is comprehensive enough to encompass any new medical finding or yet-to-be-discovered disease and yet retain an unequivocal approach to successful treatment. The revival of Ayurveda within a modern context can provide that approach. This is because Ayurveda, applied through the theory of the *tridosha* has the irrefutable capacity to rejuvenate and unify all branches of medical science— including biochemistry, physiology, pharmacology, pathology, medicine, surgery, nutrition, and psychiatry as we now know them.

Holistic health is the modern name for the wine of ancient Vedic knowledge in a new bottle. Holism is an eternal concept of the essential unity of life and the inevitable relatedness of all systems through the agency of nature.

Healing means the achievement of internal and external balance and harmony with the laws of nature. No system of medicine except Ayurveda will work universally. The basic theories of Ayurveda are universally applicable because they are a science, not just of medicine, but of the entire process of conscious living, the science of life itself.

Any accurate examination of our modern system of health care delivery must be carried out within a pluralistic model, the apex of which is institutionalized allopathic medicine, but which also includes medicine of the popular culture in colorful profusion. In addition to board-certified internists or surgeons, Americans patronize chiropractors, nutritionists, naturopaths, acupuncturists, body workers, massage therapists, and psychic and religious counselors. The basis of most of these less formal disciplines is naturopathy.

---

*The recent scientific emphasis on the role of the immune system indicates that Western science may be returning to a conviction that holism is essential to the successful practice of medicine.

Naturopathy uses the traditional Ayurvedic methods to cleanse the *doshas*: water, air, sunlight, herbs, heat, diet, meditation, and massage. In the naturopathic approach, imbalances in the *doshas* are addressed without formal indentification. Using Ayurvedic knowledge has always helped healers to identify imbalances in some form or another, and it will continue to do so in the future.

Holistic health begins with preventive health education. Americans spend millions of dollars each year in an attempt to control and counteract the effects of accumulated doshas. For example, alcohol is often used and abused because it has a heating/liquifying tendency that increases kapha and pitta dosha and reduces vata dosha, an effect which will tend to control the "nerves" that are a sign of accumulated vata. Tobacco is used not only because it is addictive but also because it has a drying/lightening tendency which reduces Kapha dosha. Drug abuse such as addiction to tranquilizers and stimulants may originate in a physiological need to control accumulated imbalance in all three doshas. Diet pills and medications are used in a largely unsuccessful attempt to control accumulated body weight or kapha dosha. Ayurveda can provide better ways of correcting and controlling physiological imbalances. In a large segment of our population health problems are caused by faulty attitudes toward preventive health and improper education regarding basic hygiene. It is never too late to begin the process of education, although for optimal effect it should be done in the early years by both family and professional health educators. The incorporation of Ayurvedic health principles in health education at the most basic community level would produce significant cost reduction and improvement in quality of health care for individuals, institutions, and governments. Even though stress-related disorders arise from improper living, and the process of treating these disorders requires an obvious effort on the part of the health practitioner, the introduction of Ayurvedic health principles can provide for an increased rate of cure among the general popularion.

According to Ayurvedic theory, there is an important subtle consideration that determines the outcome of the cure. The *Charaka Samhita* says that all diseases are caused by at least one of three separate factors:

1. Intellectual pride or blasphemy that results in illness

2. Seeing, hearing, touching, smelling, and tasting that which is disease-producing

3. Stress due to climate, environment, or season (Ayurveda advises that diet and habits be adjusted at the juncture point of each season, for it is at the juncture of the seasons that diseases are thought to originate)

In the execution of therapy, *Charaka* says that four things are required for a successful cure, of which one is absolutely essential. The first three are:

1. The proper attitude on the part of the patient (a sincere desire to become well)

2. The proper attendant or health professional to provide care and support during the healing process

3. The proper medicine prepared and administered in the proper manner (This is the Vedic discipline of *upashaya,* the beneficial administration of medicine, diet, and health practices in order to effect a complete balancing of the *doshas*)

The combination of all these elements is important but, without the fourth ingredient, *Charaka* advises, no cure can be obtained. *The last and essential requirement is the healing awareness of an Ayurvedist or health practioner.* Even if the other three are optimally present, no cure will take place without the application of the evolved awareness of the physician or healer who has been trained to treat the immortal Self in all patients.

In Ayurvedic terms, all disease is directly equated with negativity or imbalance, and is treated exactly as if it were a personified manifestation of suffering. The Ayurvedist is trained to see the disease and the patient as separate entities and to treat the immortal Self *(purusha)* and the body it inhabits with great gentleness, but to be merciless toward the negative energy that is the disease.

Awareness through education is the great weapon of the Ayurvedist, for both *Charaka* and *Sushruta* reveal the chilling fact that disease can only come upon us when we are unaware, and that illness comes upon human beings invisibly, "like a reflection slips into a mirror." This is why Ayurveda emphasizes awareness or pure consciousness, which destroys ignorance. Ayurveda recommends deep meditation (currently best-researched and time-tested being the Transcendental Meditation and TM-Sidhi program) to establish a deep awareness of the Self that cannot be shaken.

Ayurveda is not just a compendium of herbal recipes; it is *sruti,* revealed knowledge about immortality that will be useful as long as there are people on earth. Ayurveda provides answers that are always true, just as the sun always rises at dawn and sets at dusk. Just so, heat and oil always subside *vata dosha*; cold and moisture always subside *pitta dosha*; and heat and drying or friction always subside *kapha dosha* in the body.

The most knowledgeable health practitioners recognize the need for a comprehensive, universal medical paradigm in the West, even though they may not know exactly how to locate it or translate it into modern terms. They realize that the future of our civilization is dependent upon it. With the revival of Ayurveda, they will wish to know the theory of the *tridosha* and the Vedic science upon which it is based. If we understand the laws of nature we can work within them. Whatever is against the laws of nature does not exist for long; Ayurveda supports all the laws of nature.

The Berkeley Holistic Health Center Handbook affirms the above by asserting:

> *In the future the well-being of mankind will depend to a large extent on the successful education of consumers and professionals alike. Perhaps now there is a need for a truly comprehensive system, a new conceptual model of understanding, diagnosis, prevention, and treatment of illness to be achieved by means of education.*

The creation of a new paradigm is a scientific victory, but the overthrow of an old one is a human victory. The reinstatement of the universal paradigm of Ayurveda is a victory for both science and humankind.

The Ayurvedist, as healer, has surrendered to the enormous and invincible force of nature that directs our ever-changing relative existence in all its aspects, and which ensures by virtue of its power the orderly and creative functioning of all life. The Ayurvedist relies on the laws of nature to uphold the process of evolution. The Ayurvedist is a representative of the beneficial forces of nature that arise from the unified field, the Self, and wields by virtue of right living the healing and transforming power of nature. The action of this calling is like a powerful, inevitable, upward current that carries with it all that comes within its path.

This work is fundamentally humanitarian. Others before us working within the Vedic tradition, have shared this same aspiration, as will others who come after.

INVOCATION

I rejoice that here before Dhanvantari
The blessed Lord of Immortality,
I offer you Bharat's free chief and sage,
The treasured lore from a most ancient age.
The lore of healing that makes happy and whole
Disease-infested body, mind and soul.
Thus I do pass the torch lit long ago
That you may spread its glow afar and throw
Its shining light upon the anguished heart
Of man. This the mission and this the art.
                    Shri Maharani Gulabkunverba

C H A P T E R   9

AYURVEDA, ENLIGHTENMENT AND IMMORTALITY

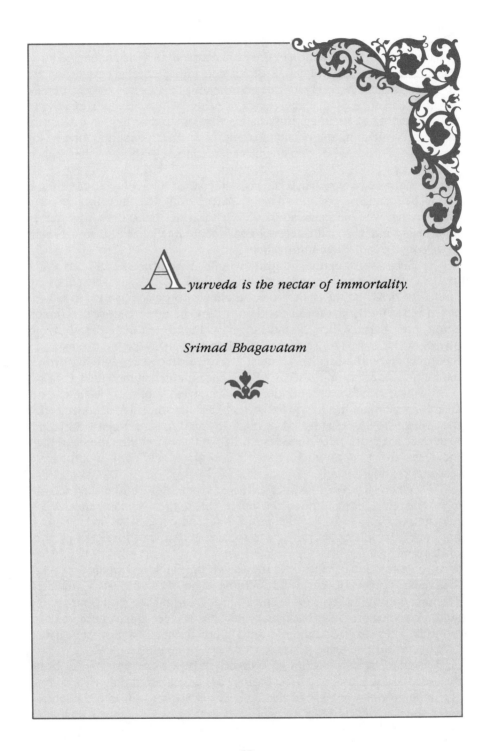

Ayurveda is the nectar of immortality.

Srimad Bhagavatam

There is a legend from the history of the *Veda* that describes the birth of Danvantari, the incarnation of the ideal Ayurvedic physician. It is said that Danvantari was born holding a vessel containing pure Ayurvedic nectar *(amrita)*. This nectar had been created from the churning of an ocean of milk by the gods and another race of ancient beings who were collaborating to find the means of attaining immortality. A great struggle to gain control of the vessel containing the nectar of immortality finally ended in victory for the Gods. It is said that by drinking this Ayurvedic nectar the gods then gained immortality.

Certainly immortality has been a goal for all people at all times, a natural desire and part of human nature. Intrinsically we believe that by living long enough we could gain all that life has to offer us. Ayurveda addresses immortality and defines it as a certain physiological refinement that will result from contact with the immortal Self.

Successfully participating in the refinement process that leads to immortality requires a clear understanding of Vedic science, the science of the unified field. When the immortal continuum of pure consciousness is contacted and infused into the mind and body through the practice of deep meditation, then balance, health, and longevity are infused into the mind and physiology. It makes sense that, if we desire longevity or life extension in the direction of immortality, we must first establish contact with that which has infinite longevity and perfect balance, the immortal unified field, the Self.

Ayurveda recommends deep meditation as the primary technique for attaining maximum health and longevity. After this fundamental contact with the unified field is established through meditation on a regular basis, the Ayurvedic literature recommends first the *panchakarma* therapies and then the herbal *rasayanas*, which may be incorporated into daily, monthly, and seasonal routines.

When all the various approaches of Ayurveda are undertaken according to the priorities mentioned, we will be able to incorporate them successfully into our lives and enjoy the results. If for some reason we had to choose only one principle of Ayurveda, it is recommended we choose the priority of deep meditation.

Restoration of balance of the *doshas* through deep meditation is the Ayurvedic approach to health through the angle of consciousness, the Self. Through the angle of education and behavior, by utilizing the agency of the mind, Ayurveda promotes balance through proper diet, and hygiene, in daily, monthly, and seasonal routines. A third Ayurvedic angle to promote balance is rejuvenation through Ayurvedic treatment programs.

All of the approaches of Ayurveda exist for one purpose: to bring the individual to a state of perfect balance or perfect health where life is lived in the complete awareness of the Self. This is Self-realization or enlightenment, the state of Unity Consciousness that is the highest state of human evolution on earth. The state of enlightenment must be cultured and maintained by a balanced and healthy physiology, one that is free of the possibility of disease. This is real health.

Many health professionals are content with the concept that health is merely the absence of disease. Ayurveda defines health as the lively presence of the unified field in the body, mind and consciousness, and declares that it is this which establishes balance of the *doshas* and prevents disease from developing. Absence of contact with the unified field will allow imbalances to occur in mind and body and subsequently allow disease to develop.

Of all the areas of research, the field of consciousness and immortality is the most rewarding and engrossing. More research needs to be conducted by the various branches of modern science on the possibilities of immortality based on the knowledge available in Vedic and Ayurvedic literature.

The main challenge for scientific research in Ayurveda is to demonstrate how biological aging can be reduced or eliminated with the application of Ayurvedic principles. If the body, mind, and consciousness are brought into balance with the eternal unified field, which has been discovered by physics to be the home of all the laws of nature, then it is indeed possible to prove with standard measurements that the body's aging has been reduced by that systematic contact with the non-changing unified field. (See the appendix to this book for research data on this subject.)

Biological measurements indicate that signs of reduced aging are now being seen when any or all of the several Ayurvedic approaches are applied. Even more exciting than this research are the results being experienced by those fortunate people who are applying Ayurvedic principles to their lives.

We have all experienced the immortal Self in some way or another. Most of us intuitively know that the gift of life is the gift of consciousness. We can be taught to systematically experience pure consciousness, the unified field, or the Self. This is the primary gift offered us by Ayurveda.

Both aspects of life, the continuum of change and the continuum of the eternal unified field against which it is reflected, are harmonized through the principles of Ayurveda. Ayurveda supports life and enables us to achieve and maintain balance. Through time, Ayurveda refines the physiology to converge upon the immortal, non-changing unified field. This means the retardation or reversal of the biological aging process with the end result of infinite life extension.

All of life is in unity whether or not we experience it as such. The Vedic knowledge, expressed as *rishi* (the knower or subject), *devata* (process of knowing or process of observation), and *chhandas* (the known or object), shows us the functioning of unified consciousness. When there is complete balance in life, complete health, the entire process of *rishi, devata* and *chhandas,* is naturally perceived as the eternal continuum of the immortal Self.

Whether the intellect is creating a multiplicity in life by conceptualizing a separation between *rishi, devata,* and *chhandas,* or whether the intellect is conceptualizing a unity of the three-in-one, it is still the "one" of the unified field that is the empirical reality of life and the source of all intellectual concepts and multiplicity.

Ayurveda offers us an opportunity to establish perfect physiological balance and health, to bring us complete awareness of the Self, ultimately culminating in a refined perception of everything in life as the Self. This is the great purpose of Ayurveda, to prepare every individual to enjoy permanently established Unity Consciousness.

The magnificent scope of Vedic science offers us fulfillment of all desires on every level of life. For this reason our human fascination with Vedic science, which is the science of ourselves and of our lives as sentient beings, will continually draw us on to further evolution, will continually draw us on by infinite reassurances to the ultimate realization that the immortality of the Self—the beauty and perfection that is living consciousness—will never, never end.

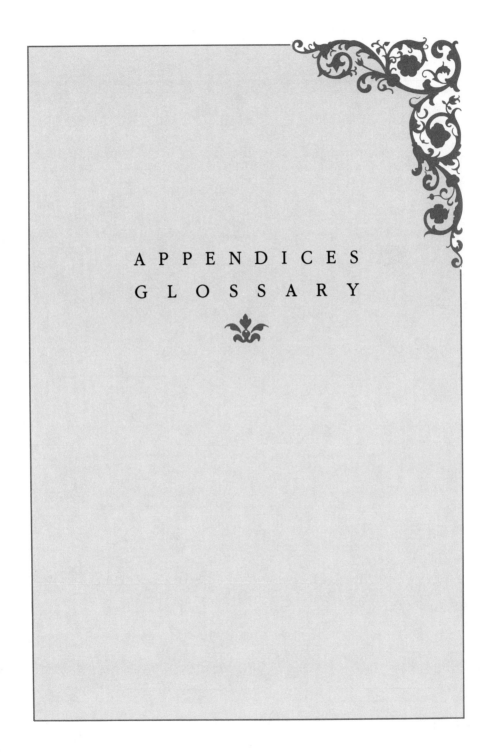

APPENDICES
GLOSSARY

APPENDIX A

SUMMARY OF SOME CURRENT RESEARCH ON THE PRINCIPALS OF AYURVEDA

The following research indicates studies that support the effects of health and longevity on individuals practicing Ayurvedic principles. The primary principle of Ayurveda is contact with the Unified Field, through the technique of deep meditation. Research is included that demonstrates the health benefits of this primary Ayurvedic principle.

REDUCED HEALTH INSURANCE UTILIZATION THROUGH THE TRANSCENDENTAL MEDITATION PROGRAM

Research being conducted at Maharishi International University, Fairfield, Iowa, by David Orme-Johnson, Ph.D., indicates that the Transcendental Meditation (TM) technique which previous research has shown to produce a unique state of deep rest, is helping to reduce the health insurance utilization and thereby health insurance costs of those participants in the group offered by Sidha Corporation International (SCI), a major insurance group of Iowa. The participants studied include approximately 1800 individuals whose only membership requirement is the regular practice of the Transcendental Meditation technique. SCI rates were lower than other insurance groups for both major categories of health care, in-patient and out-patient, in the categories of medical and surgical, but were similar to other groups for obstetrics. This pattern of less utilization due to illness suggests that the SCI group was healthier than the norm. In addition, the SCI group showed a much lower rate of increase in health care utilization as a function of age than comparison groups, supporting the findings of previous research that the TM program improves health and slows biological aging.

This study may represent an especially important finding for businesses who provide group insurance for their employees and desire to reduce growing health care costs.

SCIENTIFIC RESEARCH ON AYURVEDA
Robert Schnieder, M.D.

Although Ayurveda is several thousand years old, the Maharishi Ayurveda Prevention Program has only been available for scientific study/investigation here in the West for less than two years. So far in that time, several scientific studies have been completed, have preliminary data, or are in progress.

The aspect of Ayurveda dealing with the mind—the Transcendental Meditation and the TM-Sidha Program—have been extensively researched in over 300 published scientific studies over the past fifteen years. These results indicate significant improvements in mental, physical, behavioral and environmental health. Many of these changes are opposite to those commonly found/associated with the aging process. In fact, biological age has been found to decrease with continued practice of the TM technique. These results are in accord with the ancient/classical predictions of Ayurveda.

In the first research on the Maharishi Ayurvedic Prevention Program (MAPP), 150 unselected patients were studied for changes in health symptoms. In this group, there was a 97 percent improvement rate in one or more major health areas compared to controls. There were statistically significant improvements in energy/vitality, appetite and digestive patterns, well-being, strength/ stamina, state of mind and emotions, previous complaints, and signs of increased youthfulness (Figure A-1). In a second research study, it was found that several areas of mental health—anxiety, depression, fatigue, confusion, and anger—all improved in MAPP participants compared to matched control subjects (Figure A-2).

In a pilot study on biological aging in the Maharishi Ayurvedic Preventive Center (MAPC) participants, an average reduction of five years of biological age was documented after eight months of the MAPP.

Studies at the Massachusetts Institute of Technology are now ongoing on the Ayurvedic food supplements called *rasyanas*. Preliminary results demonstrate prevention of age-related changes in vital organs in animals.

There are many parallels being discovered between modern science and the ancient science of Ayurveda. For example, a recent scientific study found that the modern classification of Type A coronary-prone behavior, which is about twenty years old, correlates with Ayurvedic constitutional/body typing which has been in use for over 5000 years. There are also modern biophysical and brain-wave correlates of the Ayurvedic constitutional types (see Figures A-4 through A-7). This knowledge may be extremely useful for predicting which types of individuals will respond to which kinds of medical treatment and fulfills a great need in modern health care.

The preceding summarizes some of the scientific research on Ayurveda done recently in the United States. Internationally, there have been several hundred scientific studies published on Ayurveda.

In conclusion, Ayurveda has been substantially studied scientifically. With the revival of widespread interest in Ayurveda, there is now a great deal more research on Ayurveda currently in progress.

FIGURE A-1
HEALTH BENEFITS

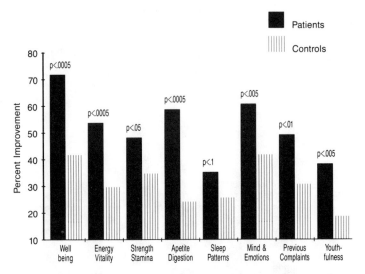

This study shows the effects of the Maharishi Ayurveda Panchakarma Program on several categories of health symptoms in 157 patients as compared to 65 control subjects who did not participate in the rejuvenation treatment but who were given an educational program on Ayurveda. The findings indicate highly significant improvements in almost all categories with the Maharishi Ayurveda Prevention Program.

Reference: R.H. Schneider, K. Cavanaugh, H.S. Kasture, S. Rothenburg, R.E. Averbach, R.K. Wallace, Eighth World Congress of the International College of Psychosomatic Medicine, Chicago, Illinois, U.S.A., September 1985.

FIGURE A-2
IMPROVED MENTAL HEALTH WITH
THE MAHARISHI AYURVEDA
PREVENTION PROGRAM

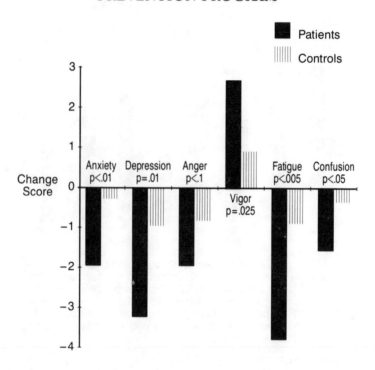

FIGURE A-3
RELATION OF TYPE A BEHAVIOR TO AYURVEDIC PSYCHOSOMATIC TYPE

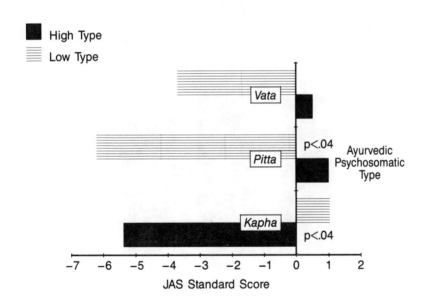

FIGURE A-4
PHYSIOLOGICAL CORRELATES
OF AYURVEDIC
PSYCHOSOMATIC TYPES:
PULSE RATE

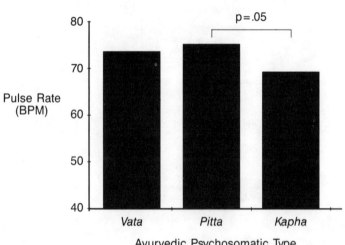

FIGURE A-5
BIOCHEMICAL CORRELATES
OF AYURVEDIC
PSYCHOSOMATIC TYPES:
PULSE RATE

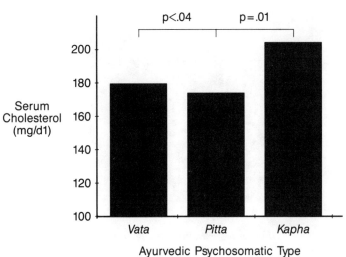

FIGURE A-6
BIOCHEMICAL CORRELATES
OF AYURVEDIC
PSYCHOSOMATIC TYPES:
TRIGLYCERIDES

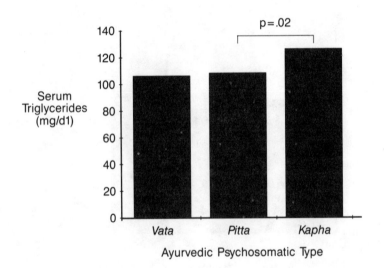

FIGURE A-7
AYURVEDIC
PSYCHOSOMATIC TYPES:
WHITE BLOOD CELLS

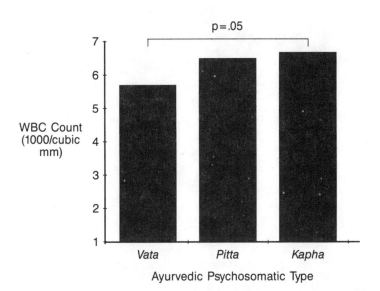

Ayurvedic Psychosomatic Type

THE EFFECTS OF THE TRANSCENDENTAL MEDITATION AND TM-SIDHI PROGRAM ON THE AGING PROCESS

ROBERT KEITH WALLACE, MICHAEL DILLBECK, ELIHA JACOBE
and BETH HARRINGTON

*Department of Biology and Psychology, Maharishi International University,
Fairfield, Iowa 52556*

FIGURE A-8
DIFFERENCE BETWEEN CHRONOLOGICAL AGE AND BIOLOGICAL AGE (Years)

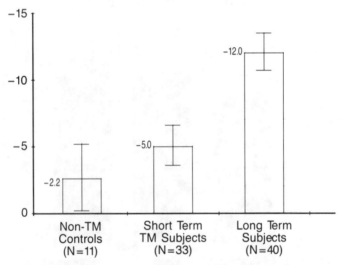

FIGURE A-8. Mean and standard error for the difference between biological age and chronological age by group, unadjusted for diet. One-way ANOVA, $F(2,81)=8.30$, $p<0.01$, $w^2=0.144$.

Reprinted from Intern. J. Neuroscience, 1982, Vol. 16, pp. 53–58. ©1982 Gordon and Breach
Science Publisher, Inc.

DISCUSSION

The results indicate that the long-term TM meditators have significantly younger mean biological age than short-term mediators, controls, and norms for the general population, and the strength of this effect is related to the length of practice of the TM technique. Further statistical analysis indicated that while subjects who excluded red meat did have younger biological ages (these were also TM participants), the effect of the TM program was independent of diet; however, the diet effect was not significant when convarying for months of TM participation. A longitudinal study involving random assignment of subjects would help to clarify the effects of preselection, attrition, and also diet.

Several previous studies have demonstrated short and long term changes as a result of the TM technique (Wallace, 1970; Wallace *et al.,* 1971; Orme-Johnson & Farrow, 1977; Benson & Wallace, 1972a, 1972b; Jevning *et al.,* 1978a, 1978b; Cooper & Aygen, 1979; Glueck & Stroebel, 1978; Wilson *et al.,* 1975). More recent studies, as mentioned before, on the advanced TM-Sidhi program have correlated the magnitude of these physiological changes with the subjectively reported experience of "pure consciousness" (Orme-Johnson *et al.,* 1981; Farrow & Herbert, 1981). The results of these and other cross-sectional studies have led different researchers to suggest that the experience of the TM and TM-Sidhi programs and their accompanying physiological state affect central nervous system functioning and this in turn influences physical and mental performance.

For example, it has been suggested that there is reduction in sympathetic tone as a result of the TM technique which leads to reduction in high blood pressure (Wallace *et al.,* 1971; Benson & Wallace, 1972a). It has also been suggested that better performance on perceptual measures as a result of the TM and TM-Sidhi program are a result of an enhancement of signal to noise ratio in information processing in the central nervous system (Clements & Milstein, 1976; McEvoy *et al.,* 1980). Greater autonomic stability found in TM participants has been suggested as the basis for faster recovery from stressful stimuli (Orme-Johnson, 1973; Goleman & Schwartz, 1976).

While the precise physiological mechanisms involved need to be further elucidated, the findings of this and other studies suggest that the experience of the TM and TM-Sidhi program affects the aging of specific autonomic and sensory processes and thereby results in significantly younger biological ages in long-term meditators.

PHYSIOLOGICAL AND PSYCHOLOGICAL CORRELATES OF AYURVEDIC PSYCHOSOMATIC TYPES

R.H. Schneider, MD., D. Orme-Johnson, Ph.D., J. Kesterson, MS, R.K. Wallace, Ph.D., Depts. of Physiology and Psychology, Maharishi International University, Fairfield, Iowa, 52556, USA.

The purpose of these studies was to determine if the classical Ayurvedic system of individual typing could account for a range of differences in physiological and psychological parameters.

Ayurveda is the main traditional system of health from India. It employs a precise system of psychosomatic typing which is based on predefined physical and mental characteristics. This typing employs the concepts of three fundamental governing properties or "doshas" in the body. According to classical descriptions, "Vata" represents properties of movement, lightness, dryness, and tendency towards anxiety. "Pitta" represents heat, metabolic processes, tendency to anger and hostility. "Kapha" represents structure, solidity, unctuousness, physical and mental steadiness.

In Study I, we attempted to correlate the Type A coronary-prone behavior pattern and its opposite, Type B, with Ayurvedic types. Thirty-seven male and female subjects were administered the Jenkins Activity Survey for Type A behavior [TAB] and clinically rated for Ayurvedic type by a standardized, semi-quantitative protocol involving history and physical examination. The results showed that high TAB was associated with high Pitta score [$p < .05$]. Kapa scores were associated with Type B behavior, and with lower scores on the subscales of speed and impatience and job involvement [$p < .05$]. Pitta plus Vata had addictive effects in predicting TAB [multiple = .40, $p < .05$].

In Study II, 150 subjects had blood sampled for several biochemicals and were clinically rated for Ayurvedic type. Kapha correlated with cholesterol levels [$r = .2$ to $.3$, $p < .01$] and triglycerides [$r = .2$ to 3, $p < .03$]. These lipids tended to be lower in Pitta and Vata types [$p < .1$].

In Study III, 17 subjects were studied for the correlation of EEG amplitude and frequency with Ayurvedic type. Kapha was correlated with higher amplitude, slower frequency EEG [$r = .46$ and $.55$, $p < .05$] - indicating a slow and relaxed type. Vata was associated with the low amplitude EEG of activation [$r = -.48$, $p < .05$]. A score for "balance" of the doshas, which reflected self-reported physical and mental health, was strongly correlated with higher amplitude EEG [posterior region, $r = 56$, $p < .02$].

These results suggest that Ayurveda offers a broad classificatory system which is associated with a wide range of physiological and psychological parameters in predicted directions. Ayurveda may contribute new insights to account for individual differences in physiological and psychological patterns.

Presented at the Eighth World Congress of the International College of Psychosomatic Medicine. Chicago, USA, 5 September, 1985.

IMPROVEMENTS IN HEALTH WITH THE MAHARISHI AYURVEDA PREVENTION PROGRAM.

R.H. Schneider, M.D., K. Cavanaugh, Ph.D., S. Rothenberg, M.D., R. Averbach, M.D., R.K. Wallace, Ph.D., Maharishi International University, Fairfield, Iowa 52556, U.S.A.

The objective of the present research was to investigate in a modern setting the classical predictions of Ayurveda, the main traditional system of medicine of India. Ayurveda focuses on prevention of disease, preservation of health, and promotion of longevity. Recently, a number of these procedures have become available for study in the West through Maharishi Ayurveda Medical Centers (MAMC).

In the first exploratory study (I), 150 consecutive participants in a MAMC were tested with a self-report health symptom instrument after completion of a 1–2 week MAMC program. This program consisted of examination for Ayurvedic constitutional type, an Ayurvedic panchakarma program of specialized massage, heat and elimination therapies, and Ayurvedic food supplements. Twenty-five control subjects were tested after participating in a didactic class on Ayurveda. For Stydy II, the Profile of Mood States (POMS) - a standardized and previously validated psychometric instrument - was administered to 62 MAMC participants before and after a 1–2 week program. The change scores were compared to 71 matched control subjects tested before and after two weeks of Ayurvedic didactic class.

The results of Study I showed that MAMC participants improved significantly (one-tailed, two-sample t-tests) on well-being ($p<.0005$), energy/ vitality ($p<.0005$), strength/stamina ($p<05$), appetite and digestion ($p<.0005$), state of mind and emotions ($p<.005$), previous complaints ($p<.01$), and signs of youthfulness and rejuvenation ($p<.005$). Sleep patterns showed marginal change ($p<.1$). In Study II, MAMC participants showed significant decreases in anxiety/tension ($p<.01$]) depression/dejection ($p = .01$), fatigue ($p<005$), and confusion/bewilderment ($p<.05$) compared to controls. Vigor/energy significantly increased ($p=.025$). Anger marginally decreased ($p=.09$).

These findings suggest that the Maharishi Ayurveda Prevention Program is associated with improvements in several areas of physical and mental health which are consistent with classical Ayurveda predictions of promotion of general health and longevity.

Paper presented at the Eighth World Congress of the International College of Psychosomatic Medicine, Chicago, USA, 7 September, 1985.

APPENDIX B

MAHARISHI AYURVEDIC MEDICAL CENTERS™ LISTING

The following is a list of the main regional centers now open for Ayurvedic treatment. We understand that eventually 50 of these centers will be opened in the United States.

MAHARISHI AYURVEDIC MEDICAL CENTER™

EAST COAST CENTER: 2112 "F" Street, N.W., Washington D.C. 20037   (202) 785-2700

MIDWEST CENTER: 3201 Middle Glasgow Road, Fairfield, Iowa 52556   (515) 472-5866

WEST COAST CENTER: 17308 Sunset Blvd., Pacific Palisades, California 90272   (213) 454-5531

GLOSSARY OF SANSKRIT TERMS

Abhaya	A variety of *harada* fruit with five sections
Abhrak bhasma	Mica or medicinal ashes of mica that requires a minimum of five years of daily preparation
Abhyanga	Medicated oil massage, a basic part of the *panchakarma* treatment
Adi Shankara	The first of original Shankara; a great Vedic scholar, interpreter of the *Veda* and founder of the Shankaracharya tradition
Agada	The branch of Ayurvedic medicine dealing with toxicology; one of eight branches of Ayurvedic medicine
Agni	The fire element; one of the five basic elements of manifest creation *(mahabhutas)*; the creative impulse of fire; digestive fire
Akasha	The space element, the finest of the five basic elements
Amla	A small, sour fruit high in vitamin C and calcium; one of three varieties of *mylobalan* fruits, the other two are *harada* and *behada*
Amrita	The nectar of immortality
Anupana	Vehicle for administering medicine; usually water, milk, clarified butter or honey
Ashtanga Hridaya	A Vedic text that means literally, "The heart of the eight-fold science of Ayurveda"
Ashwin kumaras	Literally "The horsemen," masters of the Ayurvedic tradition
Asuras	A race of ancient beings
Atharva Veda	One of the four main *Vedas*;
Atreya	A great Ayurvedist and teacher of Jivaka who was court physician to Lord Buddha
Ayana	A pathway abode or home; also, "to circulate"
Ayurveda	The science of life-extension and immortality
Ayurvedist	One who practices Ayurveda as a healing art
Ayus	Life

Badarayana	A Vedic sage also known as Krishna Dvaipayana and nicknamed "Vyasadeva," meaning the arranger or copiler of the *Veda*
Bala Vidya	The branch of Ayurvedic medicine dealing with youth or pediatrics, obstetrics and gynecology; one of eight branches of Ayurvedic medicine, bala may also mean immune system strength
Baradwaja	A Vedic sage who was elected to learn Ayurveda from Indra
Basmati	A variety of long-grain rice
Basti	One of the basic cleansing actions in Ayurveda, lubricating or medicated internal cleansing part of the five basic actions *(panchakarma)*
Behada	One of the three varieties of Indian gooseberry fruits, the other two are *alma* and *harada*
Bhagavad Gita	An important Vedic text
Bhasma	Medicinal ashes of mineral elements
Bhuta Vidya	Psychiatry, one of the eight branches of Ayurvedic medicine
Brahma	A principle cognizer of Ayurveda
Brahmacharya	The student period of life
Brahmi	An Ayurvedic herb named after Brahma in the U.S. "It is called *gotu koea.*"
Charaka	A great master of the Ayurvedic tradition who wrote the *Charaka Samhita*
Charaka Samhita	A great Ayurvedic text or encyclopedia of general medicine, still in use today
Chayavan	A recluse and celibate who upon the occasion of his marriage developed the revitalizing tonic named after him
Chayavan prash	A revitalizing tonic made of Ayurvedic herbs, named after the sage Chayavan
Churna	Finely powdered herbs
Daksha-Prajapati	A great Ayurvedic seer
Danvantari	The ideal Ayurvedic physician
Devata	The process of intellectual conception or observation in the three-in-one structure of consciousness
Dhatu	Bodily tissues; also meaning "that which supports or upholds"

Dosha	Fundamental force in physiological function; also means, "fault or break and that which becomes vitiated or deranged"
Dwiguna Makaradwaja	A medicinal compound of minerals that has been incinerated with sulfur in two succeeding operations
Ghee	Clarified butter
Grihasta	The householder or family period of life
Gunas	The three manifest tendencies of nature which are harmony (*sattva*), the spur of action or passion (*rajas*), and ignorance (*Tamas*)
Harada	One of three varieties of *mylobalan* fruits; the other two are *behada* and *amla*
Heera	Diamond
Hingula	Cinnabar
Iatrochemistry	The art of transformation of metals by using their self-referring properties; the ancient East Indian art of *rasashatra,* sometimes referred to as alchemy
Indra	A great Vedic lord who passed on the knowledge of Ayurveda to Baradwaja
Jala	The water element; one of the five basic elements (*mahabhutas*)
Jivaka	Ayurvedist and court physician to Lord Buddha; Jivaka means "living soul" or "one who gives life"
Jivataman	Living individual being; a manifestation of *purusha,* the Self
Jnana Sankalini Tantra	An ancient Vedic text
Kajali	A preliminary mineral compound used in the manufacture of *makaradwaja,* a *rasashastra* medicine
Kapha	One of the three fundamental physiological forces; the water/earth element combination described in the *tridosha* theory; a distinct constitutional or body type
Kaya	"Of the body;" one of the eight branches of Ayurvedic medicine usually described as general or internal medicine (concerns itself with diseases below the clavicle)

Kerala	A region in south India
Keshyapa	A seer of the *Veda*
Krishna Daivpayana	Also known as Badarayana, nicknamed "Vyasade-va," which means the compiler of the *Vedas*
Loha bhasma	The mineral iron prepared as a medicinal oxide
Mahabhutas	The five basic elements that make up manifest creation: earth, water, fire, air and space
Maharishi Mahesh Yogi	A great sage of the *Veda*; founder of the Maharishi Technology of the Unified Field™
Makaradwaja	A famous Ayurvedic mineral rejuvinator
Malas	Body waste products, including the hair and nails
Mandhur bhasma	Dross of molton iron prepared as a medicinal oxide
Mandukaparni	*Centella asiatica* herb, also known as "urban brahmi." Known in the U.S. as gotu koea.
Mantra	Purposeful resonance, a word whose effect is unknown.
Mukta	Pearl
Mylobalan	The Indian gooseberry fruit
Nagarjuna	A Vedic saint who popularized the art of *rasashastra*
Nasya	A nasal treatment to remove congested *doshas* from the head area; one of the five basic actions (*panchakarma*)
Nava ratna	Nine gems; a famous Ayurvedic medicine
Neelmani	Sapphire
Ojas	Vital essence; an ultra-refined nutrient; the nutritional end product of proper digestion responsible for the maintenance of health and vitality
Panchakarma	The five basic Ayurvedic health-restoring physical therapies that mimic natural bodily cleansing functions
Panna	Emerald
Parvati	Consort of Shiva, also known as Mother Divine
Phalam	Fruit
Pishti	Finely pulverized minerals usually prepared in plant juices or rose water
Pitta	One of the three fundamental physiological forces; the fire/water elements combination described in

	the *tridosha* theory and having to do with heat, light, and transformation; a distinct constitutional or body type
Pizichilli	A warming oil treatment which primary balances *pitta dosha*
Prakriti	Nature as it manifests; also individual and unique constitutional type as determined at conception
Praval	Red coral
Prithivi	The earth element; one of the five basic elements of manifest creation (*mahabhutas*)
Purusha	The immortal Self; the knower; the unified field; pure consciousness
Rajas or Rajoguna	One of the three *gunas* (tendencies) of nature; defined as the energetic and maintaining impulse of nature; the spur to action or passion
Rajistic	Having or promoting the quality of *rajas* (the spur to action or passion)
Rasa	Taste; sap, food juice, elixir, lymph, essence, purified metal oxide, gravy or sauce; the first product of digested food that subsequently nourishes the blood and all other body tissues
Rasashastra	Ayurvedic discipline specifically concerned with the preparation of medicines from inorganic materials and which outlines sophisticated procedures for unfolding the latent medicinal values of minerals to enhance their therapeutic action
Rasayana	Ayurvedic treatment for rejuvenation of the physiology and the immune system for the purpose of life-extension and immortality; one of the eight branches of Ayurvedic medicine
Rasa Ratnakar	A text on the science of *rasashastra*
Rasa sindhur	A form of *makaradwaja* made without the use of pure gold as a catalyst
Rig Veda	The first of the four *Vedas* out of which the other three *Vedas* evolve; literally, the rhythm or intervals of the universal impulses of consciousness
Rishi	The knower; part of the three-in-one structure of consciousness; a seer or scholar who cognizes the *Veda*
Sama Veda	One of the four *Vedas*

Samhita	Wholeness or totality of natural law; also encyclopedic compendium or value of the *Veda*
Sandhi	In nature, the juncture points between day and night (the two twilights—dawn and dusk); also, in the sanskrit language, the junction point between words, and in consciousness, the junction points between waking, dreaming, sleeping and pure consciousness
Sange Yashm	Jasper
Sanskrit	The language of the *Veda;* meaning elegantly polished or well put together
Sanyasi	The complete retirement period of life
Saraswati	The impulse of knowledge or wisdom
Sattva or *Satoguna*	One of the three *gunas* or fundamental tendencies of nature; defined as the creative impulse of nature; harmony or purity
Sattvic	Having or promoting the quality of *sattva* (harmony or purity)
Shalakya	One of the eight branches of Ayurvedic medicine dealing with eye, ear, nose, throat, mouth and diseases above the clavicle
Shalya	One of the eight branches of Ayurveda dealing with major surgery; a probe or sharp instrument
Shataguna Makaradwaja	A compound medicine made from the process of 100 or 1000 separate oxidations of specific mineral compounds
Shilajit	The mineral pitch tonic of the Himilayas; literally, the destroyer of weakness
Shirodara	An herbalized oil treatment for the head area
Shiva	The impulse of creative intelligence having to do with the destruction phases of natural law; Shiva's discourse on immortality to Parvati defines the principles of *rasashastra*
Shlish	The sanskrit verb that means "to join or adhere"
Shodhana	The preliminary process of purifying metals for use as *rasashastra* medicines
Shusksma	Subtle or imperceptable to the ordinary senses
Sidha	Perfected being, or saint
Sinhalese	The language of Sri Lanka

Soma	Very popular in Vedic literature is said to be true "glue of the universe." Soma can be understood as something like a fluid substance or impulse of creative intelligence which connects body and mind, physical existence and consciousness.
Sri Lanka	An Island country in the Indian ocean off the southern coast of India
Sruti	Revealed knowledge
Sthula	Gross; obvious to the ordinary senses
Sushruta	A great Ayurvedist who wrote the Sushruta Samhita
Sushruta Samhita	An encyclopedia of Ayurveda dealing mainly with surgery and toxicology
Swedana	Medicated Ayurvedic steam treatment; part of the *panchakarma* treatment
Takashila	An ancient Vedic city
Tamas and *Tamoguna*	One of the three *gunas* and fundamental tendencies of nature; defined as the retarding or destructive tendency of nature; inertia or ignorance
Tamasic	Having or promoting the quality of *tamas*
Tap	The sanskrit verb meaning to produce heat or to burn
Tola	A weight measurement equal to approximately 10 grams
Tridosha theory	(Or, the theory of the Tridhatu) According to Ayurveda, the explanation of the functioning of three basic elements known as *Kapha, pitta* and *vata* (water, fire and air) and how they operate in human physiology; the principle theory of Ayurveda
Trikantmani	Amber
Triphalla	Literally means three fruits; the famous Ayurvedic panacea that contains the three *mylobalan* fruits, *amla, harada* and *behada,* which are all varieties of the Indian gooseberry
Udhvarnta	A dry friction massage used to reduce dullness or heaviness in the body
Upanishads	Ancient Vedic texts
Upashaya	The proper and beneficial manner of administration of medicine

Upa Vedas	Near to the *Veda*; a subsidiary or subordinate part of the *Veda*; Ayurveda is considered to be an *Upa Veda*
Va	The sanskrit verb — to move
Vagbhatta	One of the great scholars of Ayurveda; Charaka, Sushruta and Vagbhatta are the three "oldies"
Vaidyas	Ayurvedic physicians; literally, "those who have knowledge"
Vajikarana	The Ayurvedic science of revitalization; one of the eight branches of Ayurvedic medicine
Vamana	Emetic therapy to cleanse the stomach area of accumulated *doshas*; one of the five basic actions (*panchakarma*)
Vanaprastha	The semi-retirement period of life
Vasant kasamakar ras	A combination Ayurvedic medicine made with herbs and minerals and used for revitalization treatment
Vata	One of the three fundamental physiological forces; the air/space element combination described in the *tridosha* theory dealing with energetic activation or nerve force; a distinct constitutional or body type
Vayu	The air element; one of the five basic elements of manifest creation *(mahabhutas)*
Veda	The cognized record of pure consciousness and its manifestations, the "blue print" of the universe
Vedic	Having to do with the knowledge of the *Vedas*
Vid	The sanskrit verb root meaning "to know"
Virechana	Purgation treatment for cleansing of accumulated *doshas* from the area of the small intestine; one of the five basic actions *(panchakarma)*
Visakyana	An identity of the same substance possessed of seemingly different qualities
Vyasadeva	The affectionate nickname given to Badarayana (Krishna Dvaipayana) which means "the arranger or compiler of the Veda"
Yajur Veda	One of the four main vedas
Yakut	Ruby
Yoga Sa'taka of Nagarguna	A collection of recipes for Vedic herbal cures

A Word From the Publisher . . .

CELESTIAL ARTS is the publisher of many excellent books on health and wellness, with an emphasis on topics of awareness such as rebirthing, meditation, consciousness, and miracles.

Among our finest publications are books by Sondra Ray, Virginia Satir, Jerry Jampolsky, Richard Moss, Barry Stevens, and Bob Mandel.

For a complete list of our books, please write or call for our free catalog.

Celestial Arts
P.O. Box 7327
Berkeley, CA 94707

(415) 524-1801

A Word From Ten Speed Press . . .

In 1983 CELESTIAL ARTS joined the publication program of the publishing house TEN SPEED PRESS. TEN SPEED's list includes career and life guidance books, fine cookbooks, and books on bicycling, outdoors, gardening, and historical reprints. TEN SPEED's list includes Don Ardell's *High Level Wellness* and Ryan & Travis' *The Wellness Workbook*. Please write or call for their free catalog.

Ten Speed Press
P.O. Box 7123
Berkeley, CA 94707

(415) 845-8414